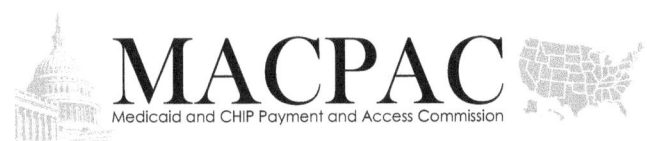

The Medicaid and CHIP Payment and Access Commission (MACPAC) was established in the Children's Health Insurance Program Reauthorization Act of 2009, and its charge was later revised in the Patient Protection and Affordable Care Act of 2010. Appointed by the U.S. Comptroller General, the 17 Commissioners have diverse backgrounds, offer broad perspectives on Medicaid and CHIP, and represent different regions across the United States.

The Commission is a non-partisan, federal, analytic resource for the Congress on Medicaid and CHIP. MACPAC is the first federal agency charged with providing policy and data analysis to the Congress on Medicaid and CHIP, and for making recommendations to the Congress and the Secretary of the U.S. Department of Health and Human Services on a wide range of issues affecting these programs. The Commission conducts independent policy analysis and health services research on key Medicaid and CHIP topics, including but not limited to:

- eligibility, enrollment, and benefits;
- payment;
- access to care;
- quality of care;
- interactions of Medicaid and CHIP with Medicare and the health care system generally; and
- data development to support policy analysis and program accountability.

As required in its statutory charge, the Commission will submit reports to the Congress on March 15 and June 15 of each year. As applicable, each member of the Commission will vote on recommendations contained in the reports. The Commission's reports provide the Congress with a better understanding of the Medicaid and CHIP programs, their roles in the U.S. health care system, and the key policy and data issues outlined in the Commission's statutory charge.

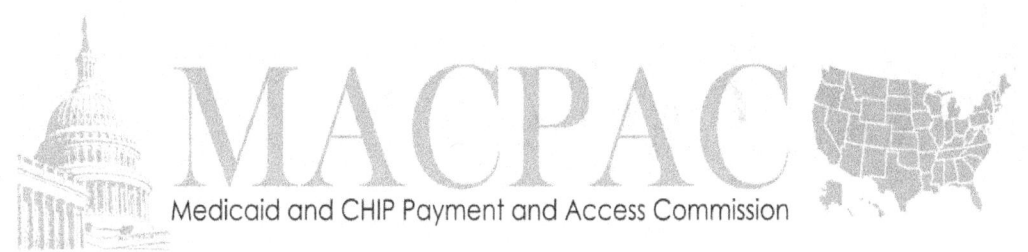

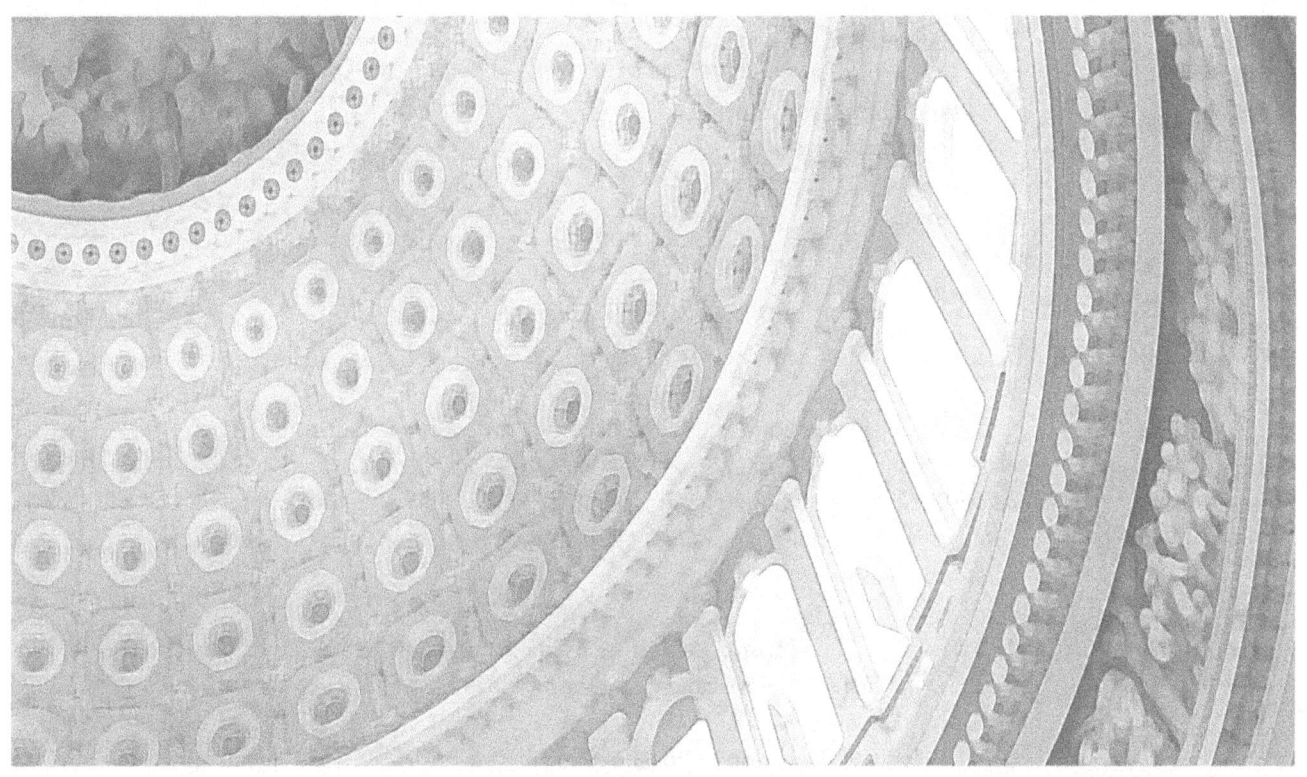

Report to the Congress on Medicaid and CHIP

March 2013

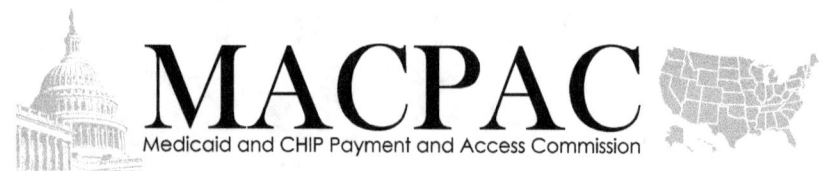

1800 M Street, NW
Suite 350 N
Washington, DC 20036
Phone: (202) 273-2460
Fax: (202) 273-2452
www.macpac.gov

Commissioners

Diane Rowland, ScD,
Chair

David Sundwall, MD,
Vice Chair

Sharon Carte, MHS
Richard Chambers
Donna Checkett, MPA, MSW
Andrea Cohen, JD
Burton Edelstein, DDS, MPH
Patricia Gabow, MD
Herman Gray, MD, MBA
Denise Henning, CNM, MSN
Mark Hoyt, FSA, MAAA
Norma Martinez Rogers, PhD, RN, FAAN
Judith Moore
Trish Riley, MS
Sara Rosenbaum, JD
Robin Smith
Steven Waldren, MD, MS

Anne L. Schwartz, PhD,
Executive Director

March 15, 2013

The Honorable Joseph R. Biden, Jr.
President of the Senate
U.S. Capitol
Washington, DC 20510

The Honorable John A. Boehner
Speaker of the House
U.S. House of Representatives
U.S. Capitol
H-232
Washington, DC 20515

Dear Mr. Vice President and Mr. Speaker:

On behalf of the Medicaid and CHIP Payment and Access Commission (MACPAC), I am pleased to submit this congressionally mandated *Report to the Congress on Medicaid and CHIP*. As outlined in our authorizing statute, MACPAC is a non-partisan Commission established to conduct objective policy and data analysis to assist the Congress in overseeing and improving these programs.

This report, the Commission's fifth since its inaugural report in 2011, is delivered to the Congress as the federal government and states are working to implement the Patient Protection and Affordable Care Act (ACA) while improving Medicaid and CHIP for the people already enrolled. In 2013, key priorities for program administrators include implementing Medicaid eligibility provisions; managing the policy and operational interactions among Medicaid, CHIP, and coverage through new health insurance exchanges; and pursuing delivery system and payment innovations for individuals dually enrolled in Medicare and Medicaid, who are among the highest need and highest cost enrollees in both programs. This report advances MACPAC's work for the Congress in these areas.

There are a number of eligibility issues among Medicaid, CHIP and coverage through health insurance exchanges that present challenges for program administrators. The Commission examined those issues and offers recommendations to the Congress to address how the programs will interact. If enacted, the recommendations would improve enrollment stability and better align a current Medicaid program known as Transitional Medical Assistance with new provisions enacted by the ACA. As implementation of the ACA continues to unfold, MACPAC will look at broader interactions among Medicaid, CHIP and exchange coverage for potential program improvements.

This report also continues the Commission's work on persons dually eligible for Medicare and Medicaid, a group that is of great interest to the Congress because of the complexity and cost of their needs. To improve service delivery and moderate costs, the Commission highlights the necessity of pursuing policy approaches that are targeted to the subpopulations covered by both Medicare and Medicaid. Medicaid payment for Medicare cost sharing is also examined in this report, including results from a new MACPAC analysis that examines states' Medicaid payment policies for Medicare cost sharing and interactions with Medicare bad debt policy. And, the report explores how Medicaid pays managed care plans for dual-eligible enrollees, an important issue as more states seek to enroll persons covered by both Medicare and Medicaid in these plans.

As in each of our reports, this report includes the Medicaid and CHIP Program Statistics (MACStats) supplement, which provides national and state-level data on enrollment, spending, health and characteristics of Medicaid and CHIP populations and Medicaid managed care. Data and information on the Medicaid and CHIP programs can be difficult to find and are spread across a variety of sources. MACStats brings those sources together and offers additional program information that is most relevant to Medicaid and CHIP policymakers today.

We hope that this report and the ongoing analytic work of the Commission will inform and assist the Congress in identifying ways to strengthen Medicaid and CHIP to assure high quality and cost-effective care for enrollees.

Sincerely,

Diane Rowland

Diane Rowland, ScD
Chair

Enclosure

Commission Members and Terms

Diane Rowland, Sc.D., Chair
Washington, DC

David Sundwall, M.D., Vice Chair
Salt Lake City, UT

Term Expires December 2013

Sharon Carte, M.H.S.
South Charleston, WV

Andrea Cohen, J.D.
New York, NY

Herman Gray, M.D., M.B.A.
West Bloomfield, MI

Norma Martínez Rogers, Ph.D., R.N., F.A.A.N.
San Antonio, TX

Sara Rosenbaum, J.D.
Alexandria, VA

Term Expires December 2014

Richard Chambers
Palm Springs, CA

Burton Edelstein, D.D.S., M.P.H.
New York, NY

Denise Henning, C.N.M., M.S.N.
Ft. Myers, FL

Judith Moore
Annapolis, MD

Robin Smith
Awendaw, SC

David Sundwall, M.D.
Salt Lake City, UT

Term Expires December 2015

Donna Checkett, M.P.A., M.S.W.
Hartford, CT

Patricia Gabow, M.D.
Denver, CO

Mark Hoyt, F.S.A., M.A.A.A.
Phoenix, AZ

Patricia Riley, M.S.
Brunswick, ME

Diane Rowland, Sc.D.
Washington, DC

Steven Waldren, M.D., M.S.
Kansas City, MO

Commission Staff

Anne L. Schwartz, Ph.D.
Executive Director

Office of the Executive Director

Amy Bernstein, Sc.D.

Mary Ellen Stahlman, M.H.S.A.

Analytic Staff

Benjamin Finder, M.P.H

Moira Forbes, M.B.A.

April Grady, M.P.Aff.

Lindsay Hebert

Angela Lello, M.P.Aff.

Molly McGinn-Shapiro, M.P.P.

Ellen O'Brien, Ph.D.

Chris Park, M.S.

Chris Peterson, M.P.P.

Lois Simon, M.H.S.

Anna Sommers, Ph.D.

James Teisl, M.P.H.

Operations and Management

Ricardo Villeta, M.B.A.
Deputy Director of Operations, Finance, and Management

Mathew Chase

Benjamin Granata

Ken Pezzella

Eileen Wilkie

Acknowledgements

The Commission would like to thank the following people who provided valuable guidance in the development of the March 2013 *Report to the Congress on Medicaid and CHIP*.

The Commission was fortunate to receive insight from staff of the U.S. Department of Health and Human Services, the Congressional Budget Office, the Medicare Payment Advisory Commission, and the Government Accountability Office regarding this report. We would like to specifically thank Christine Aguiar, Karyn Kai Anderson, Susan Anthony, Melanie Bella, Sharon Donovan, Tim Engelhardt, Jean Hearne, Jessica May, Christie Peters, Jennifer Ryan, and Carlos Zarabozo for their contributions.

We also received indispensible feedback from several state Medicaid officials, including Nancy Atkins, Pat Casanova, Jerry Dubberly, Darin J. Gordon, Cindi B. Jones, Scott Leitz, and MaryAnne Lindeblad.

Several research and policy experts provided the Commission with technical feedback, including Deborah Bachrach, Tricia Brooks, Randall Brown, Cheryl Camillo, Rob Damler, Richard Frank, Todd Gilmer, Elizabeth Hargrave, Sandra Hunt, Stephen Kuncaitis, Ethan Levy-Forsythe, Debra Lipson, John Lovelace, Jeff McCartney, Billy Milwee, Shamis Mohamoud, Patricia Nemore, Christine Nye, Jessica Nysenbaum, Frank Scalzo, Abha Shrestha, Ellen Singer, Benjamin Sommers, Michelle Kitchman Strollo, James Verdier, Shinu Verghese, and Tianne Wu.

Finally, the Commission would like to thank Lynette Bertsche, Jason Coats, Imelda Demus, and their colleagues at NORC at the University of Chicago for their assistance in editing and producing this report.

Table of Contents

Commission Members and Terms vii

Commission Staff ix

Acknowledgements xi

Executive Summary 1

Chapter 1: Setting the Context 9
    Implementing the Patient Protection and Affordable Care Act 12
    Addressing Growth in Program Spending 13
    Analysis to Frame and Support Congressional Decisions 14
    Looking Forward 15
    References 17

Chapter 2: Eligibility Issues in Medicaid and CHIP: Interactions with the ACA 19
    ACA Provisions Affecting Medicaid and CHIP Eligibility 23
    Churning 26
        Effects of churning 28
        State approaches to address churning and its effects 29
    Commission Recommendation 32
    Transitional Medical Assistance 35
        Background 36
        TMA in 2014 37
    Commission Recommendation 38
    Endnotes 40
    References 41

Chapter 3: The Roles of Medicare and Medicaid for a Diverse Dual-Eligible Population 45
    Characteristics of Dual Eligibles 49
    Medicare's Role for Dual Eligibles 49
        Why do people with Medicare need Medicaid? 49
        How do people with Medicare qualify for Medicaid? 50
    Medicaid's Role for Dual Eligibles 52
    Dual Eligibles' Service Use and Spending across Both Programs 55
        Dual-eligible subgroups 55
        Variation in spending across dual-eligible subgroups 58
        Aggregate program spending by subgroup 64
    Looking Forward 65
    Conclusion 67
    Endnotes 68
    References 69

MACStats: Medicaid and CHIP Program Statistics 71
Overview 74

Chapter 4: Medicaid Coverage of Premiums and Cost Sharing for Low-Income Medicare Beneficiaries 127
Overview of Medicare Savings Programs 130
    Medicare Savings Programs 130
Role of States in Medicare Savings Program Eligibility and Enrollment 135
    Eligibility 135
    Enrollment 138
States' Role in Determining Payment for Medicare Coinsurance and Deductibles 139
    History of lesser-of payment policies 139
Inventory of State Medicaid Payment Policies for Medicare Coinsurance and Deductibles 141
    Medicare bad debt payment 146
    Data limitations regarding Medicaid payment of Medicare coinsurance and deductibles 147
Policy Implications 147
Endnotes 149
References 150

Chapter 5: Issues in Setting Medicaid Capitation Rates for Integrated Care Plans 153
Overview of Rate Setting for Medicaid Managed Care 156
    Capitation rate development 156
    Challenges in Medicaid rate setting for dual eligibles 158
Current Experience with Managed Care for Dual-Eligible Enrollees 158
    State arrangements with dual-eligible special needs plans 159
    Program of All-inclusive Care for the Elderly 161
Medicaid Payment in the Financial Alignment Demonstrations 163
    Joint rate-setting process 163
    State examples 164
Issues for Consideration 165
    Accounting for voluntary enrollment 167
    Need for LTSS risk adjustment models 168
    Need for measures of functional status 169
    Treatment of supplemental payments 169
Endnotes 170
References 170

Appendix 173
Acronym List 175
Authorizing Language from the Social Security Act (42 U.S.C. 1396) 179
Commission Votes on Recommendations 187
Biographies of Commissioners 189
Biographies of Staff 195

List of Figures

FIGURE 2-1.	Medicaid and Exchange Coverage for Parents and Childless Adults, 2014	24
FIGURE 3-1.	Dual Eligibles, by Age, 2007	49
FIGURE 3-2.	Average Medicare Spending per All-Year, Full-Benefit Dually Eligible Beneficiary, by Type of Service, 2007	50
FIGURE 3-3.	Dual Eligibles by Medicaid Benefit Status, 2011	51
FIGURE 3-4.	Eligibility Pathways of All-Year, Full-Benefit Dual Eligibles, 2007	52
FIGURE 3-5.	Medicaid Expenditures for Dual Eligibles, 2007	53
FIGURE 3-6.	Dual Eligibles, by Length of Enrollment and Type of Eligibility, 2007	57
FIGURE 3-7.	Distribution of All-Year, Full-Benefit Dual-Eligible Enrollment, by Type of LTSS Use, 2007	57
FIGURE 3-8.	Average Medicare and Medicaid Spending per All-Year, Full-Benefit Dual Eligible, by Subgroup, 2007	58
FIGURE 3-9.	Distribution of Spending by Program and Type of Service, 2007	60
FIGURE 3-10.	Percentage of All-Year, Full-Benefit Dual Eligibles Using Selected Services, by Subgroup, 2007	61
FIGURE 3-11.	Percentage of All-Year, Full-Benefit Dual-Eligible HCBS Waiver Participants Using Selected Medicare- and Medicaid-Financed Services, by Age, 2007	63
FIGURE 3-12.	Average Medicare and Medicaid Spending per All-Year, Full-Benefit Dual Eligible Using Institutional Services, by Age, 2007	64
FIGURE 3-13.	Distribution of All-Year, Full-Benefit Dual Eligible Enrollment and Total Program Spending by Subpopulation, 2007	65
FIGURE 3-14.	Total Spending of the Highest-Cost Dual Eligibles to Medicaid, 2007	66
FIGURE 4-1.	Number of Medicaid Programs Using Lesser-of, Full-Payment, and Other Crossover Policies, 2012	142
FIGURE 4-2.	Crossover Policies for Hospital Inpatient Services, by State, 2012	144
FIGURE 4-3.	Crossover Policies for Hospital Outpatient Services, by State, 2012	144
FIGURE 4-4.	Crossover Policies for Skilled Nursing Facilities, by State, 2012	145
FIGURE 4-5.	Crossover Policies for Physician Services, by State, 2012	145
FIGURE 4-6.	State Crossover Payment Policies over Time, 1997–2012	146

List of Boxes

BOX 2-1.	Examples of Churning	29
BOX 3-1.	MedPAC's Recent Reports on People Who Are Dually Eligible for Medicare and Medicaid	54
BOX 3-2.	Methodology for the Analysis of the Dually Eligible Population	56
BOX 4-1.	Examples of Medicaid Payment for Medicare Cost Sharing	140

List of Tables

TABLE 2-1.	States Providing Continuous Eligibility to Children	32
TABLE 3-1.	Medicare and Medicaid Spending per All-Year, Full-Benefit Dual Eligible, by Type of Service, 2007	59
TABLE 4-1.	Medicare Fee-for-Service Cost-Sharing Amounts for Part A and Part B Services, Calendar Year 2013	131
TABLE 4-2.	Medicaid Benefits by Dual-Eligible Category	132
TABLE 4-3.	Legislative Milestones in Medicaid Coverage of Premiums and Cost Sharing for Low-Income Medicare Beneficiaries	136
TABLE 4-4.	Lesser-of, Full-Payment, and Other Crossover Policies, by State, 2012	143
TABLE 5-1.	Comparison of Massachusetts and Ohio Medicaid Capitation Rate Elements in Memoranda of Understanding (MOUs) for the Financial Alignment Demonstrations	166

Note: MACStats tables are listed separately on pages 72 and 73.

Executive Summary

As part of its statutory charge, each March the Medicaid and CHIP Payment and Access Commission (MACPAC) reports on significant issues affecting Medicaid and the State Children's Health Insurance Program (CHIP), two federal-state programs that play significant and growing roles in the nation's health care system. In fiscal year (FY) 2012, Medicaid financed care for an estimated 72.6 million people, over a fifth of the U.S. population, at a cost of $435.5 billion. CHIP served 8.4 million children in FY 2012, with spending of $12.2 billion.

The Commission's March 2013 *Report to the Congress on Medicaid and CHIP* focuses on several key congressional priorities including interactions between Medicaid, CHIP, and the new health exchanges and issues related to individuals who are dually eligible for Medicaid and Medicare. The report is divided into five chapters and a statistical supplement:

- Chapter 1: Setting the Context
- Chapter 2: Eligibility Issues in Medicaid and CHIP: Interactions with the ACA
- Chapter 3: The Roles of Medicare and Medicaid for a Diverse Dual-Eligible Population
- Chapter 4: Medicaid Coverage of Premiums and Cost Sharing for Low-Income Medicare Beneficiaries
- Chapter 5: Issues in Setting Medicaid Capitation Rates for Integrated Care Plans
- MACStats: Medicaid and CHIP Program Statistics

The Commission is charged with making recommendations to the Congress, the Secretary of the U.S. Department of Health and Human Services, and the states on a wide range of issues affecting Medicaid and CHIP. This report includes two recommendations related to eligibility, both of which address the changed context within which Medicaid and CHIP will function when major provisions of the Patient Protection and Affordable Care Act (ACA, P.L. 111-148 as amended) go into effect in 2014.

Chapter 1: Setting the Context

Medicaid and CHIP are at a critical juncture in their evolution. The ACA, although not fully implemented, is already changing integral aspects of Medicaid and CHIP.

Medicaid is on the cusp of a major eligibility expansion that will heighten its role as a major purchaser of health services. At the same time, the Congress will be considering the future of CHIP in the context of both the Medicaid expansion and the subsidized coverage that will be offered through health insurance exchanges.

While preparing for the changes mandated by the ACA, Medicaid and CHIP are also responding to broader issues in the health care system. These include continued growth in health care spending, a desire to enhance program efficiency and promote better health care outcomes, and pressures with respect to the financing and delivery of long-term services and supports (LTSS).

Chapter 1 explores how these issues shape the context in which Medicaid and CHIP programs operate, focusing on how issues affecting health care in the U.S. are influencing the two programs.

Chapter 2: Eligibility Issues in Medicaid and CHIP: Interactions with the ACA

To increase the number of Americans with health insurance, the ACA created a continuum of coverage by expanding Medicaid eligibility, providing new premium tax credits for the purchase of private health insurance, and instituting numerous other changes effective in 2014. The design of the ACA specifically changes some aspects of Medicaid and CHIP as well as creates a new environment within which these programs operate. Chapter 2 makes recommendations related to two specific interactions between the ACA and the Medicaid and CHIP programs.

The ACA expands Medicaid eligibility in 2014 (effectively at state option, based on a 2012 Supreme Court decision) to nearly all adults with income up to 138 percent of the federal poverty level (FPL). Other ACA policies that streamline eligibility, enrollment, and renewal processes will increase insurance coverage of individuals who were previously eligible but not enrolled. The Congressional Budget Office projects that Medicaid and CHIP enrollment will increase by 8 million people in 2014 because of the ACA.

While states may choose not to expand coverage to low-income adults, in 2014 all states must implement other ACA changes to streamline eligibility determinations and to standardize income-counting methodologies across states and programs. In addition, states can no longer require face-to-face interviews for low-income applicants, can only schedule regular redeterminations every 12 months, and cannot require families to provide information already available to the state.

Churning, the phenomenon of individuals enrolling and disenrolling from different sources of health insurance over a relatively short period of time, is a long-standing problem in Medicaid and CHIP and can create barriers to access for enrollees as well as administrative burdens for providers, plans, payers, and states. While some ACA policies may mitigate churning, they will not eliminate it. Millions of individuals may continue to move between sources of coverage—or off of coverage altogether—when required to report what are typically modest income changes.

In the past, some state Medicaid programs have implemented a policy known as 12-month continuous eligibility to help reduce churning. Such policies allow individuals to enroll for a full year regardless of changes in family income or composition. Twelve-month continuous eligibility is an explicit statutory option for children in Medicaid, and states have flexibility under existing rules to implement 12-month continuous eligibility for adults in Medicaid and in separate CHIP programs. However, this flexibility may no longer be available for some Medicaid and CHIP enrollees in 2014 as an unintended consequence of implementing the modified adjusted gross income requirements.

To retain states' authority to implement 12-month continuous eligibility and in order to mitigate some of the hazards associated with enrollment churning, the Commission recommends:

> **Recommendation 2.1:** In order to ensure that current eligibility options remain available to states in 2014, the Congress should, parallel to the existing Medicaid 12-month continuous eligibility option for children, create a similar statutory option for children enrolled in CHIP and adults enrolled in Medicaid.

Enactment of the ACA also creates new questions about Transitional Medical Assistance (TMA). TMA provides additional months of Medicaid coverage to millions of families who might otherwise become ineligible and uninsured due to an increase in earnings from employment. While TMA has been a provision of Medicaid law for nearly 40 years, states face perennial uncertainty about whether it will continue to be funded.

In states expanding to the new adult group, TMA may no longer be necessary to prevent uninsurance and could create unnecessary confusion and administrative burden for enrollees and eligibility workers. If states implementing the adult group expansion could opt out of TMA because of the presence of other coverage options, states would save money.

In the interest of promoting administrative simplification—for enrollees, providers, and payers, including the federal and state governments—and maximizing continuity of coverage and care, the Commission recommends:

> **Recommendation 2.2:** The Congress should permanently fund current Transitional Medical Assistance (TMA) (required for six months, with state option for 12 months), while allowing states to opt out of TMA if they expand to the new adult group added under the Patient Protection and Affordable Care Act.

Chapter 3: The Roles of Medicare and Medicaid for a Diverse Dual-Eligible Population

Individuals who are dually eligible are low-income seniors and persons with disabilities who are enrolled in both Medicare and Medicaid. In 2011, there were 10.2 million dual eligibles, including 7.5 million people with Medicare who qualified for full Medicaid benefits and 2.7 million partial-benefit dual eligibles, for whom Medicaid paid only for Medicare premiums or cost sharing. Annual Medicaid spending on dual eligibles exceeds $100 billion.

Persons dually eligible for Medicare and Medicaid are a diverse group, including people who are young and old, people who are relatively healthy as well as those who are gravely ill, and people who have no disabling or chronic conditions as well as those with significant disabilities. LTSS use accounts for the majority of Medicaid spending for dual eligibles but utilization varies from full-time nursing home residents to those who do not use any Medicaid LTSS. The diversity of the population is reflected in its widely varying use of services and spending.

Chapter 3 describes the care needs and patterns of service use and spending among several subgroups of the dually eligible population, to better inform the design of policy solutions that take into account this diversity. The Commission plans to continue examining options for improving care and services for dual eligibles and the implications for both Medicare and Medicaid.

Characteristics of dual eligibles. The majority of dually eligible individuals are adults age 65 and older who qualify for Medicare on the basis of their entitlement to a Social Security retirement benefit; other dual eligibles are under age 65 and are enrolled in Medicare as a result of a serious disability.

Among all-year, full-benefit dual eligibles, 59 percent had no LTSS use in 2007 and 41 percent used some LTSS, including 19 percent who used institutional services in Medicaid, 10 percent who used Medicaid home and community-based waiver services as an alternative to institutionalization, and 11 percent who used Medicaid state plan LTSS only.

Average annual Medicare and Medicaid spending varied widely across these four subgroups, from $70,000 for people who used institutional services in Medicaid to about $15,000 for people who did not use any LTSS.

Medicare's role for dual eligibles. For all dual eligibles, Medicare is the primary source of health insurance, covering physician services, inpatient and outpatient hospital care, post-acute care, and prescription drugs. Full-benefit dual eligibles who do not use LTSS rely, on average, almost exclusively on Medicare. These individuals account for 59 percent of all-year, full-benefit dual-eligible enrollees but just 11 percent of Medicaid spending on those dual eligibles.

Medicaid's role for dual eligibles. Medicaid provides financial assistance with Medicare costs for poor and near-poor Medicare beneficiaries, as well as access to services not covered by Medicare, including LTSS, behavioral health services, vision, dental care, and other wraparound services.

People who need an institutional level of care (who used Medicaid institutional LTSS or waiver services) rely much more heavily on Medicaid and account for the majority of Medicaid spending on all-year, full-benefit dual eligibles (78 percent).

A small number of high-need, high-cost beneficiaries account for most Medicaid spending for dual eligibles. The highest-cost 10 percent to Medicaid account for roughly half of all Medicaid spending on all-year, full-benefit dual eligibles.

Chapter 4: Medicaid Coverage of Premiums and Cost Sharing for Low-Income Medicare Beneficiaries

The Medicare program was originally designed to serve eligible individuals without regard to their income and includes beneficiary cost-sharing requirements such as premiums, deductibles, and copayments similar to private health insurance. From its earliest days, Medicaid covered some of the costs of medical care for low-income Medicare beneficiaries, but many persons eligible for this assistance did not enroll.

Out of concern that low-income individuals would forgo needed care when faced with cost-sharing requirements beyond their means, the Congress enacted a series of provisions to make Medicaid's role in paying for these costs explicit and to encourage greater enrollment. Today, there are four Medicare Savings Programs (MSPs), each with different income and asset-level requirements.

The Commission is examining MSPs as part of its ongoing analytic agenda related to individuals who are dually eligible for Medicaid and Medicare, as well as its longstanding interest in Medicaid payment policy. It seeks to better understand the interaction between the Medicaid and Medicare programs at the state level, and, ultimately, whether such interactions affect access to services for dually eligible individuals.

Chapter 4 describes the MSPs and mechanisms by which Medicaid contributes to the costs of medical care for low-income Medicare beneficiaries. These include payment of Medicare premiums, coinsurance payments, and deductibles for low-income persons who meet certain income and asset thresholds. Some low-income persons qualify for full Medicaid coverage for services that are not covered by Medicare.

While federal requirements set minimum standards for MSP eligibility and benefits, states vary in the methods used to determine MSP eligibility and the eligibility levels for full Medicaid benefits. As a result, MSP enrollment rates vary among states. The MSPs covered 8.3 million dual eligibles in 2011.

States have a certain amount of flexibility in how they pay for Medicare cost sharing, but current state policies have not been readily available at the federal level. For this report, MACPAC reviewed publicly available state policies in order to develop an up-to-date and complete picture of how states pay for these cost-sharing amounts. The study looked at payment policies for four provider types: inpatient hospitals, outpatient hospitals, skilled nursing facilities (SNFs), and physicians. State policies were classified into three categories:

- Full payment: the state pays the full amount of Medicare deductibles and coinsurance, regardless of the Medicaid payment rate.
- Lesser of: the state pays the lesser of the full Medicare deductible and coinsurance or the difference between the Medicaid rate and amount already paid by Medicare.
- Other: the state policy does not clearly fall into either of the above categories.

Most states use lesser-of policies, with 36 states using these policies for hospital inpatient and outpatient services, and 39 states using them for SNF and physician services. It also appears that there has been a substantial shift toward use of the lesser-of policy since it was explicitly authorized in the Balanced Budget Act of 1997 (P.L. 105-33). Thirteen states pay full cost sharing for inpatient hospital services, 12 states pay full cost sharing for skilled nursing facilities, and 11 states pay full cost sharing for outpatient hospital and physician services.

Medicare cost-sharing payment policies can vary within a state. About half of the states have a lesser-of policy for all four provider types and four states have a full-payment policy for all four provider types; the remaining 18 states mix and match policies in a variety of combinations.

Medicaid payments for acute care, which includes Medicaid services not covered by Medicare as well as Medicare coinsurance and deductibles, are estimated at $21.4 billion, or 20 percent of Medicaid spending for all dual eligibles in 2007. Medicaid payments for Medicare premiums accounted for another $10.5 billion in 2007.

The Commission will continue to explore the role that states play in assuring access to services for dual eligibles, including state enrollment policies and the effect of state Medicaid payment policies for Medicare cost sharing.

Chapter 5: Issues in Setting Medicaid Capitation Rates for Integrated Care Plans

Persons who are dually eligible for both Medicare and Medicaid are among the highest-need and highest-cost individuals in both programs. Several states are serving dual eligibles through risk-based care models and many are working with the Centers for Medicare & Medicaid Services (CMS) to develop more effective integrated care models.

The approach to setting Medicaid capitation rates for plans participating in these programs will be a key factor in determining whether the initiatives move forward, are sustained over time, and meet expectations for financial savings. Chapter 5 focuses on several policy and technical issues related to setting appropriate Medicaid capitation rates for integrated care programs serving dual eligibles.

Overview of rate setting for Medicaid managed care. Medicaid capitation rate-setting methods vary from state to state, although most follow the same general process. States begin with a baseline of historical claims and eligibility data and make adjustments to reflect expected costs. Capitation rates are set for groups of enrollees to reflect differences in predicted service use for each group. States may further refine their payment methodologies to mitigate financial risk and to create incentives related to performance and quality.

Ideally, the capitation rates should be set at levels that are neither so low that plans avoid enrolling individuals with the greatest needs or limit access to services, nor so high that there are no incentives for plans to be efficient. The biggest challenge in setting capitation rates for dual eligibles is properly accounting for the cost of LTSS, which constitutes approximately 70 percent of Medicaid spending for full-benefit dual eligibles. Putting plans at risk for LTSS should create incentives for plans to provide services in the most cost-effective setting. However, as noted in Chapter 3, spending on LTSS varies widely among dual eligibles, creating substantial financial risk for plans if the needs of the enrolled population do not match the assumptions built into the capitation rates.

Current experience with managed care for dual-eligible enrollees. States have experience with two existing integrated care programs for dual eligibles: (1) state arrangements with Medicare Advantage dual-eligible special needs plans (D-SNPs) and (2) Program of All-inclusive Care for the Elderly (PACE) plans. They have used a range of rate-setting tools to create financial incentives while accounting for population differences and financial risk to the plans.

However, while risk adjustment is one of the strongest tools for states to appropriately balance incentives and risk, only a few states have implemented a Medicaid risk adjustment process for dual eligibles. Commonly used risk adjustment models are based on diagnostic data that do not reliably predict LTSS costs, and the predictive power of new models that use LTSS-related measures (e.g., frailty, functional status) has not been widely researched. Given the differences in LTSS benefits in each state, a single risk adjustment model may not accurately predict LTSS costs across states and some states may need to develop their own models.

Medicaid payment in the financial alignment demonstrations. The CMS financial alignment demonstrations seek to coordinate the Medicare and Medicaid rate-setting process to take into account cross-program interactions and share overall cost savings across both programs. The Medicare rate-setting methodology will be consistent across all participating states and will be based on the existing Medicare Advantage and Medicare Part D rate-development processes, including risk adjustment. States and their actuaries, with review from CMS, will develop the Medicaid payment rates and make separate payments to participating health plans.

Issues for consideration. As the financial alignment demonstrations and other efforts to expand risk-based models for this high-cost, high-need population move ahead, policymakers will need to consider several additional payment issues, including accounting for voluntary enrollment, the need for LTSS risk adjustment models and appropriate measures of functional status, and the treatment of supplemental payments.

MACStats: Medicaid and CHIP Program Statistics

MACStats is a standing section in all Commission reports to the Congress. In this report, MACStats includes state-specific information about program enrollment, spending, eligibility levels, optional benefits covered, and federal medical assistance percentages (FMAPs), as well as an overview of cost sharing permitted under Medicaid, and the dollar amounts of common FPLs used to determine eligibility for Medicaid and CHIP.

- Total Medicaid spending grew by only about 1 percent in FY 2012 to $435.5 billion. Total CHIP spending grew by less than 2 percent to $12.2 billion.

- The number of individuals ever covered by Medicaid grew by less than 2 percent from an estimated 71.7 million in FY 2011 to 72.6 million in FY 2012. CHIP enrollment grew from 8.2 million to 8.4 million. Few states changed income eligibility levels for Medicaid and CHIP in 2012.

- In FY 2012, federal Medicaid spending decreased and state spending increased due in part to the expiration of a temporary increase in FMAPs.

- The Medicaid and CHIP programs accounted for 15.5 percent of national health expenditures in calendar year 2011, and their share is projected to reach 20 percent in the next decade.

CHAPTER 1

Setting the Context

CHAPTER 1

Setting the Context

Medicaid and the State Children's Health Insurance Program (CHIP) play significant roles in U.S. health care, with an estimated 73 million people covered by Medicaid and 8 million by CHIP in fiscal year (FY) 2012. These individuals primarily include low-income children and their families, children and adults with disabilities, and low-income seniors. Together, these joint federal-state programs cover nearly half of the nation's children for at least part of the year, over 6 million seniors, and about 10 million persons with disabilities. In addition, reflecting the diversity of needs in the populations it covers, Medicaid provides benefits—most notably long-term services and supports (LTSS)—not typically offered (or not covered to the same extent) by other payers, including Medicare and CHIP.

As major purchasers of care, Medicaid and CHIP accounted for 15.5 percent of national health care spending in 2011. In addition to financing services for enrollees, these programs help finance the nation's health care safety net and reduce the burden of uncompensated care for certain providers (MACPAC 2013, 2011).

As MACPAC presents this report to the Congress, the fifth since its inaugural report in March 2011, Medicaid and CHIP are at a critical juncture in their evolution. The Patient Protection and Affordable Care Act (ACA, P.L. 111-148, as amended), although not fully implemented, is already changing integral aspects of Medicaid and CHIP as well as the landscape of the broader health care system. Medicaid is on the cusp of a major eligibility expansion that will heighten its role as a major purchaser of health services. At the same time, Congress is considering the future of CHIP, a program that interacts with Medicaid and, as of 2014, the subsidized coverage offered through newly created health insurance exchanges.

Continued growth in health care spending, a challenge for all payers of health services, is a major focus for federal and state policymakers charged with administration and oversight of Medicaid and CHIP. At a time of heightened concerns about state and federal budgets, this growth has created renewed pressure to pursue delivery system and payment innovations that can enhance program efficiency and promote better health outcomes. And as the baby boom generation begins to retire, Medicaid faces new pressures with respect to the financing and delivery of LTSS, for which it is the predominant payer.

In this report, MACPAC presents analyses related to four issues facing Medicaid and CHIP: (1) interactions among Medicaid, CHIP, and new exchange coverage related to eligibility, (2) the growing population of persons served by both Medicare and Medicaid (referred to as dual eligibles), (3) Medicaid policies for payment of Medicare premiums and cost sharing, and (4) improving Medicaid payment methodologies for integrated care plans that combine acute care and long-term services and supports. This chapter explores how these issues fit into the larger context of Medicaid and CHIP program improvements, focusing on how issues affecting health care in the U.S. are influencing the two programs.

Implementing the Patient Protection and Affordable Care Act

At its enactment in 1965, Medicaid initially offered coverage to low-income families with children, persons with disabilities or blindness, and seniors. Over the years, the Congress has made numerous changes to the program in terms of eligibility, covered services, and financing. In addition, CHIP was enacted in 1997 to offer health coverage to many low-income children who were uninsured at that time. While smaller than Medicaid in terms of enrollment and spending, CHIP has had a great impact on uninsurance for children: while 22.8 percent of children were uninsured in 1997, only 9.7 percent were uninsured in 2012 (Martinez and Cohen 2012).

Implementation of the ACA will be one of the most fundamental changes in Medicaid since its enactment. The ACA has the potential to expand Medicaid eligibility in 2014 to nearly all adults with income up to 138 percent of the federal poverty level (FPL, $15,856 for a single person in 2013), and is expected to expand Medicaid and CHIP coverage by 8 million people in 2014—most of them low-income adults (CBO 2013a, CBO 2013b).

Even in states that choose not to expand Medicaid coverage, the coordination of eligibility and enrollment systems among Medicaid, CHIP, and the exchanges is also expected to increase the enrollment of individuals into Medicaid and CHIP for those who were previously eligible but not enrolled in the programs. This is sometimes referred to as the "woodwork" or "welcome mat" effect.

The ACA also creates a federal subsidy program for individuals not eligible for Medicaid but with income below 400 percent FPL to purchase health insurance through health insurance exchanges. For Medicaid and CHIP, the existence of exchange coverage will create new market dynamics with potentially wide-ranging effects on individuals, providers, and health plans, as well as states and the federal government.

For Medicaid program administrators, implementing the 2014 eligibility expansion and managing the policy and operational interactions with exchange coverage are a high priority in 2013 (KFF et al. 2013). States are on the front line of the expansion, with numerous operational, policy, and financing issues at the forefront of their agendas. In addition to preparing to enroll a large number of new individuals, states are redesigning and upgrading information technology systems to determine eligibility and share information with health insurance exchanges; implementing new eligibility policies and procedures; and planning for longer-term funding of the expansions (NASBO 2012).

Of particular concern to policymakers is how the use of new income determination methodologies for Medicaid and CHIP will affect eligibility and enrollment. Issues of importance include the accuracy of such income determinations; the number of individuals who will move from one source of coverage to another and how frequently; and the potential impact on families whose members have different sources of coverage, including different benefits, cost-sharing requirements, and provider networks.

Addressing Growth in Program Spending

Like Medicare and private payers, Medicaid and CHIP face spending pressures. Total federal and state spending on Medicaid was $436 billion in FY 2012 (MACStats Table 6). Overall health care spending growth has moderated in recent years, and Medicaid spending grew by only about 1 percent between FY 2011 and FY 2012. Factors contributing to slower Medicaid spending growth included state efforts to slow spending, lower enrollment growth during the period, and expiration of a provision that temporarily increased the federal financial contribution for Medicaid (Truffer 2013). In FY 2012, 48 states implemented at least one Medicaid cost-control measure and 47 had plans to do so in FY 2013 (Smith et al. 2012).

However, factors including enrollment growth and the increasing cost of Medicaid benefits per beneficiary will lead to Medicaid spending growth in the coming years. Federal outlays for Medicaid are expected to rise over the next decade, from 1.8 percent of gross domestic product (GDP) in 2014 to 2.2 percent in 2023. In comparison, CBO expects Medicare to grow from 3.0 to 3.5 percent of GDP over the same period (CBO 2013b). Concerns about federal spending generally have created renewed scrutiny on all entitlement programs.

Medicaid and CHIP also account for a large and rising share of state budgets (NASBO 2012). The state share of Medicaid spending accounted for 13.4 percent of state-funded budgets in state fiscal year (SFY) 2011 (MACStats Table 15). This was up from 12 percent in SFY 2010, partly due to the expiration of the temporary increase in Medicaid funding (MACPAC 2013). Such growth is of particular concern to governors and state legislators given that states are required to balance their budgets each year.

Medicaid officials have relied on a number of blunt strategies for moderating costs, including restricting eligibility (a practice limited under the ACA), reducing or slowing the rate of growth in payments to providers, and tightly managing covered benefits. For some states, these strategies may have reached their limits. Instead, Medicaid programs are seeking better value by pursuing more creative ways to meet the health needs of the program's diverse populations while creating incentives for more efficient use of high-quality services.

This move toward prudent purchasing is not new; over the years, Medicaid and CHIP have pursued many strategies including enrolling populations into comprehensive risk-based managed care and primary care case management and implementing medical homes. Today, programs are also testing innovative payment approaches, including tying payment to health outcomes, exploring new models for bundled and global payments, and expanding the reach of risk-based managed care from low-income children and parents to populations with more extensive health care needs. The policy focus is particularly intense for the dual-eligible population, who, while accounting for a relatively small share of total Medicaid enrollees account for a large amount of program spending, particularly for LTSS (see Chapter 3). A number of states and the federal government are working together on financial alignment demonstrations that will extend the use of risk-based managed care for dual eligibles. The diversity of the dually eligible population in terms of their health needs, service use, and spending patterns, however, may suggest that careful thought and planning are needed as strategies are developed.

Analysis to Frame and Support Congressional Decisions

The policy context for Medicaid and CHIP, as well as continued pressure to ensure a sustainable path for program spending while meeting the health needs of the low-income populations served by the two programs, provide the backdrop for MACPAC's consideration of the policy issues in this report.

With a mission to assist Congress in examining Medicaid and CHIP issues and to provide evidence-based, data-driven, non-partisan information and recommendations for program improvement to the Congress, the Secretary of the U.S. Department of Health and Human Services, and the states, MACPAC has sought in this report to build on the foundational, largely descriptive work undertaken during the Commission's start-up period. The Commission's initial reports describe many key features of Medicaid and CHIP including financing and payment; access to care for children and adults; the role of managed care; a profile of services, spending, and quality measures for persons with disabilities; program integrity; and data for program management and monitoring; as well as MACStats data supplements. Building on a sound analytic foundation, the Commission looks forward to offering the Congress more in-depth analyses and recommendations going forward.

As the 113th Congress weighs the issues facing Medicaid and CHIP, this MACPAC report provides information on and analyses of four key issues as well as state-specific Medicaid and CHIP data and program information:

▶ **Medicaid and CHIP interactions with exchange coverage related to eligibility.** The expansion of Medicaid coverage to adults with incomes up to 138 percent FPL and implementation of the new income counting methodology (known as modified adjusted gross income or MAGI) raise a number of policy issues, explored in Chapter 2. For example, small changes in income may lead to individuals changing coverage between Medicaid and subsidized exchange coverage, a phenomenon known as churning. The chapter examines the extent and impact of churning and includes a recommendation to the Congress to minimize churning by permitting states to implement 12-month continuous eligibility for adults in Medicaid and children in CHIP.

Additionally, the chapter reviews the historical experience and rationale for Transitional Medical Assistance (TMA), a program that provides additional months of Medicaid eligibility for certain individuals whose incomes increase. TMA may no longer be needed, given the availability of exchange coverage with premium tax credits and cost-sharing reductions for individuals whose incomes are too high for Medicaid. The Commission makes recommendations regarding the future of TMA in the context of the Medicaid expansion.

- **Service use and spending patterns for persons dually eligible for Medicare and Medicaid.** Dual eligibles are a diverse group with service needs that vary widely. Chapter 3 examines that diversity by exploring their service use and spending based on their use of LTSS. The data confirm that a small number of enrollees with substantial need for LTSS drive Medicaid spending for full-benefit dual eligibles. This spending and service use analysis illustrates the need for delivery system and payment solutions that are targeted to specific subgroups of the dually eligible population.

- **State Medicaid policies for payment of Medicare premiums and cost sharing.** Chapter 4 examines one aspect of the interaction between Medicaid and Medicare in serving low-income individuals for whom Medicare is the primary payer: Medicaid's coverage of Medicare premiums and cost sharing. To date, there has been no single source of information on state policies for Medicaid payment of Medicare cost sharing. MACPAC undertook this analysis to better understand the array of state policies and to lay the foundation for future work on this topic including how payment policies may affect access to care for dual eligibles. The results of that work are presented here, along with details of the eligibility and benefits available to partial-benefit dual eligibles whose higher incomes qualify them for varying levels of assistance in paying Medicare premiums and cost sharing.

- **Medicaid rate setting for integrated managed care plans serving dual eligibles.** As states and the federal government continue to pursue integrated care delivery models for dual eligibles, payment adequacy and accuracy are key issues. Chapter 5 explores the details of capitation rate development and refinement for high-cost, high-need enrollees, focusing on the complexities of accounting for LTSS use.

- **MACStats.** A standing supplement to MACPAC reports, MACStats features state-specific data on Medicaid and CHIP enrollment, spending, income eligibility levels, enrollee characteristics, and other program features.

Looking Forward

MACPAC has already begun the process of analyzing issues that it will share with the Congress in June of this year and in subsequent reports. Through its own analyses of Medicaid administrative data, efforts to collect information not readily available from existing sources, consultation with states and others expert in the Medicaid and CHIP programs, and review of the research literature, MACPAC will be developing more in-depth analyses on a number of issues over the coming year, including:

- further examination of the new market created by the ACA; interactions among Medicaid, CHIP, and exchange coverage;

- new analyses of populations such as persons with disabilities and dual eligibles who have high rates of service use and spending, to inform program improvements that could lower cost growth and improve quality;

- consideration of the future of CHIP;

- analyses on supplemental payments for institutional providers;

- an assessment of Medicaid waivers;

- identification of gaps in data availability, consistency, and quality to ensure that timely information is available for program management and policy development; and

- additional attention to program integrity efforts, including developing a better understanding of the effectiveness of individual programs, how federal and state agencies are coordinating their efforts, and the impact of new program integrity activities created by the ACA—an issue particularly relevant with the substantial expansion of Medicaid in 2014.

MACPAC plans to focus special attention on the future of CHIP given that, under current law, no federal CHIP funding is available after FY 2015. Whether Congress extends CHIP funding and, if not, how children enrolled in CHIP will transition into either Medicaid or exchange coverage remains to be seen (MACPAC 2013).

The Commission also plans to spotlight the role of Medicaid and CHIP with respect to maternity care, oral health, and behavioral health. The Commission will continue work related to access to care for Medicaid and CHIP enrollees, consistent with its statutory charge. MACPAC will continue to support congressional deliberations by providing objective and data-driven analyses on these and other issues.

References

Congressional Budget Office (CBO). 2013a. *Effects of the Affordable Care Act on health insurance coverage—February 2013 baseline.* Washington, DC: CBO. http://www.cbo.gov/publication/43900.

Congressional Budget Office (CBO). 2013b. *The budget and economic outlook: Fiscal years 2013 to 2023.* Washington, DC: CBO. http://www.cbo.gov/sites/default/files/cbofiles/attachments/43907-BudgetOutlook.pdf.

Congressional Budget Office (CBO). 2012. *Estimates for the insurance coverage provisions of the Affordable Care Act updated for the recent Supreme Court decision.* Washington, DC: CBO. http://www.cbo.gov/sites/default/files/cbofiles/attachments/43472-07-24-2012CoverageEstimates.pdf.

Kaiser Family Foundation (KFF), Robert Wood Johnson Foundation and Harvard School of Public Health. 2013. *The public's health care agenda for the 113th Congress.* Washington, DC: KFF. http://www.kff.org/kaiserpolls/upload/8405-F.pdf.

Martinez, M.E., and R.A. Cohen. 2012. *Health insurance coverage: Early release of estimates from the National Health Interview Survey, January–June 2012.* Hyattsville, MD: National Center for Health Statistics. http://www.cdc.gov/nchs/data/nhis/earlyrelease/insur201212.pdf.

Medicaid and CHIP Payment and Access Commission (MACPAC). 2013. *Overview of Medicaid and CHIP.* Washington, DC: MACPAC. http://www.macpac.gov/reports.

Medicaid and CHIP Payment and Access Commission (MACPAC). 2012. *Report to the Congress on Medicaid and CHIP.* March 2012. Washington, DC: MACPAC. http://www.macpac.gov/reports.

National Association of State Budget Officers (NASBO). 2012. *State expenditure report: Examining fiscal 2010–2012 state spending.* Washington, DC: NASBO. http://www.nasbo.org/sites/default/files/State%20Expenditure%20Report_1.pdf.

Smith, V.K., K. Gifford, and E. Ellis, et al. 2012. *Medicaid today: Preparing for tomorrow—A look at state Medicaid program spending, enrollment and policy trends.* Washington, DC: Kaiser Commission on Medicaid and the Uninsured. http://www.kff.org/medicaid/upload/8380.pdf.

Truffer, Christopher. 2013. Medicaid expenditures outlook. Presentation before the Medicaid and CHIP Payment and Access Commission, January 15, 2013, Washington, DC. http://www.macpac.gov/home/meetings/2013-01.

CHAPTER 2

Eligibility Issues in Medicaid and CHIP: Interactions with the ACA

Recommendations

Eligibility Issues in Medicaid and CHIP: Interactions with the ACA

2.1 In order to ensure that current eligibility options remain available to states in 2014, the Congress should, parallel to the existing Medicaid 12-month continuous eligibility option for children, create a similar statutory option for children enrolled in CHIP and adults enrolled in Medicaid.

2.2 The Congress should permanently fund current Transitional Medical Assistance (TMA) (required for six months, with state option for 12 months), while allowing states to opt out of TMA if they expand to the new adult group added under the Patient Protection and Affordable Care Act.

Key Points

To meet the requirements of the Patient Protection and Affordable Care Act (ACA, P.L. 111-148, as amended), all states must make changes to their Medicaid and CHIP programs and will experience enrollment increases in 2014, regardless of whether or not they expand coverage to adults with incomes up to 138 percent of the federal poverty level (FPL). This chapter explores key issues states will face related to Medicaid and CHIP eligibility in the context of new ACA provisions.

- In 2014, millions of individuals may move between sources of coverage during the year, or off of coverage altogether, due to changes in income or family composition. This churning can create access barriers for enrollees and administrative and financial burdens for providers, plans, payers, and states.

- State flexibility to reduce churning by using 12-month continuous eligibility, which allows states to waive the requirement that enrollees report income changes during the year, is hampered by provisions of the ACA requiring a new income-counting methodology that is consistent across states. The Commission recommends that states continue to be able to implement 12-month continuous eligibility for adults in Medicaid and children in CHIP.

- While Transitional Medical Assistance (TMA) has helped prevent uninsurance by providing six or more months of Medicaid coverage to families whose earnings increase, states face perennial uncertainty about whether TMA will continue to be funded. To end this uncertainty, particularly for states not expanding coverage to 138 percent FPL for adults, the Commission recommends permanently funding TMA.

- In states expanding coverage for adults, TMA may no longer be necessary to prevent uninsurance and could create unnecessary confusion and administrative burden for enrollees and states. The Commission also recommends allowing states to opt out of TMA if they expand to the new adult group.

CHAPTER 2

Eligibility Issues in Medicaid and CHIP: Interactions with the ACA

To increase the number of Americans with health insurance, the Patient Protection and Affordable Care Act (ACA, P.L. 111-148, as amended) created a continuum of coverage with substantial federal funding by expanding Medicaid eligibility, providing new premium tax credits for the purchase of private health insurance, and instituting numerous other changes effective in 2014. Implementing these large-scale, complex changes will be an ongoing endeavor for the federal and state governments.

The ACA's expansion of Medicaid eligibility in 2014 to nearly all adults with income up to 138 percent of the federal poverty level (FPL), or less than $16,000 annually for an individual, is a key element of the law's projected reduction in the number of uninsured (CBO 2012). Prior to the ACA, federal Medicaid law generally did not permit coverage of childless adults who were not pregnant, disabled, or at least age 65. This expansion therefore represents a departure for many state Medicaid programs, of which only five previously provided comprehensive Medicaid coverage of childless adults through waivers approved by the Secretary of the U.S. Department of Health and Human Services (the Secretary) (KFF 2010). The ACA defined these adults as a mandatory eligibility group as of 2014. However, the Supreme Court decision in *National Federation of Independent Business (NFIB) v. Kathleen Sebelius* in 2012 allows states to forgo the expansion without facing any penalty.

Besides the expansion of Medicaid to the new adult group, other ACA policies that streamline eligibility, enrollment, and renewal processes will increase insurance coverage. Thus, many new Medicaid and State Children's Health Insurance Program (CHIP) enrollees in 2014 will be individuals who were previously eligible but not enrolled. In 2014, Medicaid and CHIP enrollment is projected to increase by 8 million people because of the ACA, with another 7 million covered through health insurance exchanges (CBO 2013a). In 2022, Medicaid and CHIP enrollment is projected to increase by 12 million people because of the ACA, with exchange plans covering another 26 million (CBO 2013b).

Eligibility for Medicaid, CHIP, and other forms of public and private coverage has important implications beyond whether or not an individual receives coverage. These programs differ in the services they cover and the cost of those services to enrollees—through premiums, deductibles, and copayments. Federal and state spending on each enrollee also differs among these programs, as well as the level and source of payments to health care providers.

In addition to the expansion to adults up to 138 percent FPL, the ACA alters Medicaid and CHIP eligibility in several ways—changes that affect all states, even those choosing not to expand Medicaid in 2014. One key provision state Medicaid and CHIP programs must implement is the ACA's new income-counting methodology—modified adjusted gross income (MAGI)—for the purpose of aligning eligibility determinations for Medicaid and CHIP with those made for subsidized coverage through health insurance exchanges. The goal of this new method is to streamline eligibility determinations and to standardize income-counting methodologies across states and programs.

The design of the ACA—an expanded Medicaid program, a continuing CHIP program, and new options for accessing private coverage—is projected to substantially decrease the number of uninsured Americans but may create new challenges. For example, small changes in income may lead to individuals switching from one program to another or a loss of insurance—a phenomenon called churning, which can create barriers to access for enrollees, and burdens on providers, plans, payers, and states. One potential solution discussed in this chapter is 12-month continuous eligibility, a current state option that may no longer be available for some Medicaid and CHIP enrollees in 2014 as an unintended consequence of implementing the MAGI requirements.

Enactment of the ACA also creates new questions about Transitional Medical Assistance (TMA), a provision of Medicaid law that has been in place for nearly 40 years. TMA provides additional months of Medicaid coverage to millions of families who might otherwise become ineligible and uninsured due to an increase in earnings or hours of employment. In 2014, however, TMA may no longer be necessary to prevent uninsurance in states where the combination of Medicaid, CHIP, and subsidized exchange coverage extends to 400 percent FPL. In fact, its continuation could create unnecessary confusion and administrative burden for enrollees and eligibility workers. If states implementing the adult group expansion could opt out of TMA because of the presence of other coverage options, states would save money by no longer paying state matching funds for TMA.

This chapter focuses specifically on the issues of churning and TMA in 2014 and the Commission's recommendations to address these issues. To set the context for these issues, the chapter first describes specific aspects of Medicaid and CHIP eligibility affected by the ACA. It then turns to a discussion of churning—its extent and impact—followed by an analysis of various policy options to address the phenomenon. The final section presents the historical experience and rationale for TMA before turning to a discussion of its relevance in the new policy environment created by the ACA.

In its analysis and formulation of recommendations on both of these topics, the Commission was guided by the principles of promoting administrative simplification—for enrollees, providers, and payers, including the federal and state governments—and maximizing continuity of coverage and care, while attempting to minimize mandatory federal and state spending.

ACA Provisions Affecting Medicaid and CHIP Eligibility

Four provisions of the ACA that will have a substantial impact on Medicaid and CHIP eligibility, described in detail below, are:

- expanded coverage to the new adult group;
- a maintenance of effort (MOE) provision to prevent states from rolling back eligibility;
- MAGI, the new method for counting income for determining the eligibility of some individuals; and
- expanded Medicaid eligibility for children.

Coverage of the new adult group. Historically, Medicaid has primarily covered low-income children, parents, pregnant women, persons with disabilities, and individuals age 65 and older. However, income limits for these individuals have varied both by eligibility group and state, with parents often having the most restrictive income requirements to qualify for Medicaid. The ACA extended coverage to adults who fit into none of these categories. As written, adults with incomes at or below 138 percent FPL are defined as a mandatory eligibility group beginning in 2014. However, the Supreme Court decision in *NFIB v. Sebelius* ruled that the federal government may not penalize non-expansion states by withholding other federal Medicaid funding.[1]

It should be noted that in many states where the expansion is implemented, both adults without dependent children and some parents of dependent children will be considered newly eligible. Current Medicaid coverage of parents, under Section 1931 of the Social Security Act (the Act), varies widely by state, with upper-income eligibility currently as low as 10 percent FPL, as shown in Table 10 of MACStats. If parents are ineligible for Medicaid under Section 1931 because their income is too high, or because their assets exceed the threshold used in some states, they will be eligible for the new adult group if their income is below 138 percent FPL, in states that implement the expansion. For example, in a state with Section 1931 levels at 50 percent FPL, parents with incomes between 51 and 138 percent FPL may be considered newly eligible and may qualify for enhanced federal financing.

States will receive enhanced federal financing to support the costs of the new adult group. For spending on individuals in the new adult group who would not have been eligible under state rules on December 1, 2009, the federal government will bear the lion's share of these costs. Specifically, the federal medical assistance percentage (FMAP), frequently referred to as the federal match, will be as follows for newly eligible individuals:

- 100 percent in 2014, 2015, and 2016;
- 95 percent in 2017;
- 94 percent in 2018;
- 93 percent in 2019; and
- 90 percent in 2020 and each year thereafter.

States that delay implementing the expansion to 138 percent FPL to the new adult group until 2017 or after would not receive a 100 percent newly eligible FMAP, because this matching rate is tied in the statute to specific calendar years.

Since April 1, 2010, states have had a statutory option to cover the new adult group with their existing FMAP. By July 2012, seven states and the District of Columbia had taken up this state plan option (KFF 2012).[2] Beginning in 2014, states may be able to receive enhanced FMAP funding for these individuals.

States are not eligible for the newly eligible FMAP until they expand to the new adult group up to 138 percent FPL. A partial expansion—for example, up to 100 percent FPL—will not entitle states to the higher matching rate (CMS 2012a). If a state decides to opt out of the expansion, childless adults and parents who otherwise would have been eligible for Medicaid beginning in 2014 may qualify instead for subsidized exchange coverage if their income is at least 100 percent FPL (Figure 2-1). If their income is below 100 percent FPL, many may not have access to federally subsidized coverage, although they would be exempt from the tax penalty for not having coverage (CMS 2013a).

Maintenance of effort. The ACA also includes an MOE provision that generally prevents states from reducing eligibility below what was in place when the ACA was enacted (March 23, 2010) until 2014 for adults and through fiscal year (FY) 2019 for children. This MOE applies even if the group had been covered at state option. According to the Centers for Medicare & Medicaid Services (CMS), the MOE does not apply if a state's waiver coverage ends and is not renewed; the MOE does not require states to extend existing waivers (CMS 2011a).

Through 2013, a state certifying that it has a budget deficit may obtain an exemption from the MOE for nonpregnant, non-disabled adults above 133 percent FPL. Three states used this authority in 2012. Hawaii reduced eligibility levels for parents and childless adults from 200 to 133 percent FPL; Illinois reduced eligibility for parents from 185 to 133 percent FPL; and Minnesota reduced eligibility levels for childless adults from 250 to 200 percent FPL (KFF 2013).

Modified adjusted gross income. MAGI is the new national income-counting methodology for subsidized exchange coverage that also applies to Medicaid and CHIP for children, their parents,

FIGURE 2-1. Medicaid and Exchange Coverage for Parents and Childless Adults, 2014

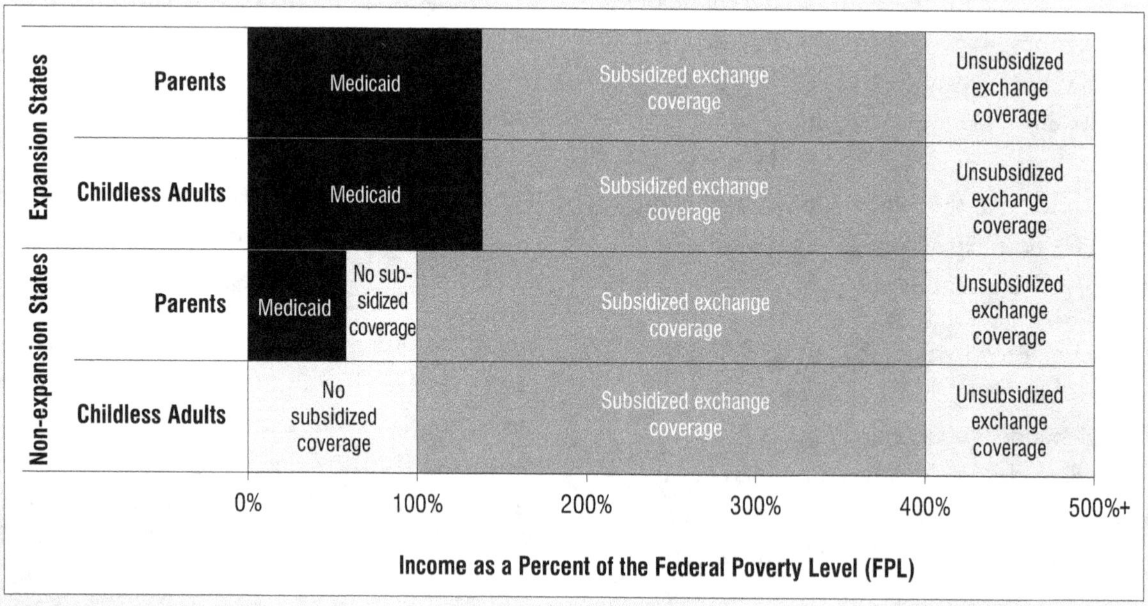

		0% – 100%	100% – 138%	138% – 400%	400% – 500%+
Expansion States	Parents	Medicaid	Medicaid	Subsidized exchange coverage	Unsubsidized exchange coverage
	Childless Adults	Medicaid	Medicaid	Subsidized exchange coverage	Unsubsidized exchange coverage
Non-expansion States	Parents	Medicaid	No subsidized coverage	Subsidized exchange coverage	Unsubsidized exchange coverage
	Childless Adults	No subsidized coverage	No subsidized coverage	Subsidized exchange coverage	Unsubsidized exchange coverage

Income as a Percent of the Federal Poverty Level (FPL)

Notes: Although states' current Medicaid eligibility levels for parents vary by state, ranging from 10 to more than 133 percent FPL in many states, the median level is 37 percent FPL; most states do not currently cover childless adults (KFF 2013). Subsidized exchange coverage is available to individuals between 100 and 400 percent FPL who are not eligible for Medicaid or CHIP; thus, in states implementing the expansion, subsidized exchange coverage will be available between 138 and 400 percent FPL. Premium and cost-sharing subsidies available through exchanges phase down as income increases.

Source: MACPAC analysis

pregnant women, and the new adult group. For these populations, MAGI is intended to reduce the variation, complexity, and confusion created by multiple methods for counting income currently used by states. All states, even those not implementing the expansion to the new adult group, are required to use MAGI in 2014, necessitating modifications to state eligibility systems and processes. Thus, conversion to MAGI as the standard methodology for counting income may be the ACA provision affecting the greatest number of Medicaid and CHIP enrollees in 2014.

When determining eligibility under current law, states have flexibility to disregard whatever sources or amounts of income they choose. Once MAGI takes effect in 2014, for those populations, the flexibility for states to achieve new expansions using income disregards goes away. Instead, only one disregard will exist under MAGI. States will be required to disregard income equal to 5 percent FPL. For this reason, eligibility for the new adult group is often referred to at its effective level of 138 percent FPL, even though the federal statute specifies 133 percent FPL.

Shifting to MAGI will significantly change how state Medicaid and CHIP programs count income. The calculation of MAGI begins with adjusted gross income, generally following the Internal Revenue Service's (IRS's) Form 1040, plus tax-exempt interest and foreign earned income. This approach will be used even for individuals who do not file a tax return.[3] MAGI includes deductions from the 1040 that have never been used in Medicaid or CHIP (e.g., educator expenses, moving expenses, student loan interest deduction). To date, there has been little federal guidance on how state eligibility systems are to incorporate deductions taken for tax purposes that have never been used in Medicaid or CHIP. In addition, MAGI excludes income that has typically been included in Medicaid and CHIP eligibility determinations, such as individuals' pretax contributions to retirement accounts. While child support has historically been counted as income for low-income families seeking Medicaid (with a disregard for the first $50 per month), MAGI excludes child support payments altogether.

Beginning in 2014, asset tests are prohibited for MAGI-based populations. While only four states currently have asset tests for children, 27 states still use them for parents (KFF 2013). For individuals not subject to MAGI (e.g., individuals eligible on the basis of being age 65 and older, disabled, or needing long-term services and supports), asset tests and states' current income-counting flexibilities continue.

In order to accommodate these changes, states are modernizing their eligibility determination systems, for which the federal matching rate is now 90 percent (CMS 2011b). As of December 2012, 49 states had received CMS approval of their plans to implement upgrades to their Medicaid eligibility systems, for which they had nearly $2.1 billion in federal Medicaid spending (CMS 2012b).

Eligibility for 6- to 18-year-olds. Although Medicaid coverage was originally available only to children receiving cash assistance, the Congress has expanded eligibility over the years to children based on income as a percentage of the federal poverty level. Currently, state Medicaid programs are required to cover children under age 6 up to 133 percent FPL, and children age 6 to 18 up to 100 percent FPL.

Effective January 1, 2014, states must extend Medicaid eligibility up to 138 percent FPL for 6- to 18-year-olds. This change will only affect the 19 states currently using separate CHIP coverage for these children.[4] In meeting this requirement, states will enroll these children in a Medicaid-expansion CHIP program—that is, these children will be enrolled in Medicaid, but the state will continue to receive the enhanced FMAP from federal CHIP funds. CHIP-funded coverage separate from Medicaid will continue to be a state option for children above 138 percent FPL.

Enrollment in a Medicaid-expansion CHIP program rather than a separate CHIP program has several implications. Children in Medicaid-expansion CHIP programs are subject to federal Medicaid benefits requirements and cost-sharing limitations, and thus are entitled to all of Medicaid's mandatory services, including Early and Periodic Screening, Diagnostic, and Treatment (EPSDT) services, generally without any enrollee cost sharing. Moreover, if a state's federal CHIP funding is exhausted, it can fall back to federal Medicaid funds at the regular Medicaid matching rate for children enrolled in a Medicaid-expansion CHIP program—an option not available for separate CHIP programs without a waiver.

Churning

The eligibility policy changes highlighted above are considerable and will result in individuals moving from Medicaid or CHIP to exchange coverage—and vice versa—as their eligibility for these programs changes. Minimizing frequent coverage changes, which have the potential to negatively affect health, costs, and administrative burden, is in the best interests of enrollees, providers, plans, and states.

Churning refers to individuals enrolling and disenrolling in different sources of health insurance, often in a relatively short period of time. Research on churning has historically focused on transitions from Medicaid or CHIP to uninsurance. For purposes of this chapter, churning is defined to also encompass enrollment transitions between Medicaid, CHIP, and subsidized exchange coverage. It should be noted, however, that even in states where the combination of Medicaid, CHIP, and subsidized exchange coverage extends to 400 percent FPL, income changes will cause many individuals to move from Medicaid to coverage without direct public subsidies. These are generally projected to be individuals whose income rises above 138 percent FPL and who have an offer of employer-sponsored insurance (ESI) considered affordable under the ACA (§1401 of the ACA, 26 CFR 1.36B-2(c)(3)(v), Buettgens et al. 2012).

As people switch between programs, churning can lead to disruptions in continuity of care if provider networks differ among programs. Likewise, churning can lead to changes in covered benefits and cost sharing. As described in greater detail below, research indicates that, under such circumstances, individuals are more likely to forgo primary and preventive care. Persons with chronic conditions or behavioral health issues are more likely than others to be affected by the disruptions that may result from churning. Delayed care may result from changes in provider networks and confusion on the part of plans, providers, and enrollees about who is covered and under which benefits package. In addition, churning may make it more difficult for plans to coordinate care effectively and can increase administrative burden and costs as individuals who were disenrolled attempt to re-enroll. Churning may also create increased administrative burden for states and the federal government as they process and track eligibility determinations for Medicaid, CHIP, and exchange coverage.

Prior research has shown that significant churning occurs during enrollees' regularly scheduled redeterminations (Fairbrother and Schuchter 2008). This is often because of administrative burdens and barriers to renewal (Czajka and Mabli 2009). While many of these individuals re-enroll within a few months, churning interrupts their coverage and is a burden to payers, providers, and plans—especially since these individuals were often eligible for Medicaid or CHIP during their period without coverage (Summer and Mann 2006). Many states have taken administrative steps to reduce churning at redeterminations, such as eliminating requirements for face-to-face interviews and using data available to the state rather than obtaining new paperwork from enrollees (KFF 2013). Several new policies to reduce churning will be required in 2014 for populations whose eligibility is assessed based on MAGI—for example, face-to-face interviews cannot be required, regular redeterminations can only be scheduled at 12-month intervals (not every six months, as in some states), and families cannot be required to provide information already available to the state (CMS 2012c).

Although churning often takes place at regularly scheduled redeterminations, a significant source of churning in 2014 may result from income changes that occur between annual redeterminations. One study estimated that within a six-month period, 35 percent of adults with incomes below 200 percent FPL would have income changes that would shift their eligibility from Medicaid to exchange coverage or the reverse; within a year, an estimated 50 percent—28 million people—would have income changes requiring a program change (Sommers and Rosenbaum 2011).

To reduce churning that occurs from income changes within a year, states have the option to implement 12-month continuous eligibility in their Medicaid and CHIP programs. This allows states to waive the requirement in federal regulations that enrollees report changes in income during the year that could affect their eligibility. It is not clear what percentage of enrollees actually report required income changes.

Extent of churning. Churning is a well-documented phenomenon in Medicaid and CHIP. In 2007, depending on the state and the size of its programs, between 11 and 67 percent of children who were enrolled in a separate CHIP program at any point during the year were also enrolled in Medicaid-financed coverage at some time during the same year (Czajka 2012). An analysis of data from the Medical Expenditure Panel Survey for 2000–2004 found that 49 percent of adults and 43 percent of children were uninsured six months after disenrolling from Medicaid (Sommers 2009).

Although the ACA creates new programs to reduce the number of uninsured, these new programs also increase the opportunity for churning between programs. Particularly in states where no eligibility gap will exist in 2014 between Medicaid, CHIP, and subsidized exchange coverage, churning between programs may be more prevalent than churning off of coverage altogether.

Shifts in coverage may not all be detrimental or inappropriate—for example, when individuals shift out of Medicaid to ESI because of a new job and an increase in income. Another example of a potentially beneficial shift in coverage may occur when a child enrolled in a separate CHIP program switches into Medicaid (if a decrease in income makes the child eligible) in order to access more generous benefits and cost sharing.

Based on the policies of the ACA, if annual redeterminations show that individuals are no longer eligible for Medicaid but are eligible for subsidized exchange coverage, they will need to switch programs. As described in greater detail below, states may be able to minimize the potential adverse effects of such transitions.

Estimates on the extent of churning in 2014. As previously mentioned, it was estimated that within a six-month timeframe, more than 35 percent of all adults with family incomes below 200 percent FPL would experience a change in income that would cause them to lose eligibility for Medicaid but gain eligibility in the exchanges, or the reverse (Sommers and Rosenbaum 2011). An estimated 50 percent of these adults (28 million) would experience a change in eligibility between the programs within one year, according to the study. This study was conducted prior to the Supreme Court's decision allowing states to forgo the expansion and thus assumed that all states would expand coverage. The authors also note that actual churning will depend on the extent to which individuals report income changes, states capture such changes, and those changes are processed to effectuate a change in enrollment. Box 2-1 provides examples of churning that could occur in 2014.

In states that forgo the expansion, the nature of churning will likely be different due to gaps in eligibility between Medicaid and subsidized exchange coverage. Consider, for example, a state where low-income parents are eligible for Medicaid up to 50 percent FPL. Because subsidized exchange coverage is only available to those with income between 100 and 400 percent FPL, an individual whose income drops from 125 to 75 percent FPL could churn from subsidized exchange coverage to having no insurance. Most states do not offer Medicaid coverage to childless adults, so many non-expansion states in 2014 may see childless adults eligible for substantial exchange subsidies between 100 and 400 percent FPL, but no coverage below 100 percent FPL.

Effects of churning

Churning may result in changes in provider networks, covered benefits, and cost sharing for enrollees. Changes in provider networks may force individuals to seek new providers or to face higher out-of-pocket costs for retaining relationships with providers that are out of network for their new source of coverage. Changes in covered benefits may result in breaks in care. Dental coverage, for example, may vary greatly between Medicaid, CHIP, and exchange coverage. Changes in cost sharing may be confusing for individuals and lead to higher out-of-pocket spending. Moving from exchange coverage to Medicaid would lead to lower out-of-pocket costs, however.

Individuals who churn may be more costly and prone to forgo preventive and primary care. A 2008 study conducted in California found that adults under age 65 who experience interruptions in Medicaid are at increased risk of hospitalizations that could have been prevented with adequate primary and preventive care (Bindman et al. 2008). Not only might this have detrimental effects on the health of the enrollee, it may be financially burdensome for states to pay for this more expensive form of treatment.

In Florida, diabetic Medicaid enrollees who experienced a brief lapse in coverage returned to the program with greater use of hospital care, including emergency room visits. As a result, average Medicaid spending on these enrollees was 75 percent higher in the three months following their re-enrollment, compared to the three months prior to their lapse in coverage (Hall et al. 2008). Similar results were also found for Medicaid enrollees with depression (Harman et al. 2007).

Churning may create additional administrative burden for states, providers, and plans. Moving back and forth between programs may involve additional paperwork and processing, which can be costly for states and plans. The amount of these increased costs is difficult to quantify, but state officials consistently report that large numbers of people disenrolling and then re-enrolling proves to be more costly than if enrollment had been stable (Summer and Mann 2006).

Interruptions in care affect quality monitoring and improvement activities. For many health care quality measures, individuals must be enrolled in the plan for 12 months. Otherwise, health care

> **BOX 2-1. Examples of Churning**
>
> **Churning between Medicaid and exchange coverage.** In 2014, Alice is a healthy 19-year-old who recently graduated from high school. She has a part-time job at a retail clothing store, where she is not offered health benefits. With her gross income of about $1,200 a month, or 125 percent FPL, she is enrolled in Medicaid. As business picks up, her manager offers her additional hours, which increases her income to about $1,400 a month, or 150 percent FPL. Because the information she has received from Medicaid clearly requires her to report any change in income that could affect eligibility, she notifies the Medicaid agency in her state. Based on this information, the state redetermines her eligibility, finding that she is eligible for subsidized exchange coverage rather than Medicaid. She churns to exchange coverage, for which she pays $60 per month out of her own pocket. Because her Medicaid managed care plan does not participate in the exchange, she must choose a new plan among the several offered in the exchange. After some research, she finds an exchange plan that includes her current primary care provider.
>
> After eight weeks of augmented hours, business wanes, Alice returns to her previous work schedule, and her income goes back to 125 percent FPL. She contacts the state Medicaid agency again and is determined eligible for Medicaid once more. Ultimately, she will be back in her previous Medicaid plan. Had 12-month continuous eligibility been available in her state, Alice could have remained in her Medicaid plan, without the state and affected health plans having to process her changes.
>
> **Churning between Medicaid and CHIP.** In 2014, Bobby is an 8-year-old Medicaid enrollee with autism who attends weekly behavior therapy sessions. He lives with his dad, who has a gross income of $1,900 a month (150 percent FPL for a family of two). His dad then begins working an additional eight hours per week, which he hopes will be permanent, increasing the family's monthly income to $2,400 (185 percent FPL). Because their state does not have 12-month continuous eligibility, Bobby's father is required to report any income changes affecting eligibility, and Bobby is now ineligible for Medicaid but eligible for CHIP. (The out-of-pocket premiums for Bobby's dad's subsidized exchange coverage will increase by approximately $60 per month to $140 per month.)
>
> In Bobby's state, the health plans available through CHIP do not include the clinic where he receives therapy. In addition, the CHIP program in his state covers fewer therapy visits than Medicaid. For additional therapy visits at the new provider they find, his dad will need to pay out of pocket. Because they cannot afford the additional therapies, even with the additional hours, Bobby's father considers reducing his hours to ensure Bobby can continue getting his therapy visits.

quality could appear poor in a plan where new enrollees need care that was preventable but was not addressed prior to their current coverage. Researchers note that individuals enrolled for less than 12 months have not been exposed to enough care to experience its health-promoting effects, thus making it difficult to assess the quality of the care they receive (Ku et al. 2009). Similarly, plans may be unwilling to seek long-term savings from care management if individuals are covered for short periods of time.

State approaches to address churning and its effects

States have experience with churning in their current programs and are exploring a number of options for minimizing the effects of churning, beginning in 2014, as individuals move among Medicaid, CHIP, and exchange coverage.

Plan requirements. Some states are taking steps in their contracts with health plans to mitigate the increased challenges that churning may pose. Massachusetts, for example, has constructed managed care contract language to ensure that enrollees receive adequate care when transitioning between programs. The state requires managed care organizations (MCOs) receiving transitioning individuals to complete a transition plan for the enrollee that is tailored to the individual's specific health care needs (Ingram et al. 2012).

States may also decide to take a multi-market approach, encouraging health insurance carriers to participate in Medicaid, CHIP, and exchange coverage. If carriers have a single plan that participates simultaneously in Medicaid and exchanges, then individuals may remain with the same insurer and network of providers when their eligibility shifts, even if their benefits and cost sharing change. A carrier may have separate plans in the Medicaid and nongroup markets but try to align the networks between the plans as much as possible, depending on factors such as providers' willingness to participate in Medicaid (Lovelace 2013). However, when carriers have separate plans in these markets, provider networks and plan payments to those providers may differ significantly between plans.

Minnesota currently requires all commercial MCOs in the nongroup market to also participate in Medicaid, but it is not clear whether this requirement will be in place in 2014 (Leitz 2013). In the 1990s, California aligned plan requirements in the Medicaid and nongroup markets so that carriers could easily participate in both, if they won contracts to do so. In both states, however, some counties run their own Medicaid managed care plan, which is often the sole source of Medicaid for residents in those counties (Leitz 2013, Finocchio 2012). Thus, in those counties, a multi-market plan may not be available even if the state has aligned plan requirements. Moreover, states may have reasons to continue contracting with Medicaid-focused plans without a multi-market presence despite the potential effects on churning—for example, if those plans have developed competencies around the unique needs of Medicaid enrollees.

Bridge plans. Tennessee proposed a specific multi-market plan approach to CMS, which would allow individuals of the same family who would otherwise have coverage under different programs to receive coverage through the same health plan. In particular, the state sought approval of having Medicaid MCOs cover Medicaid enrollees' family members who themselves are not eligible for Medicaid. This is commonly referred to as a bridge plan (Tennessee IEPI 2011). CMS has announced its support for this approach (CMS 2012a). While the exchange-eligible family member could be enrolled in the Medicaid plan, the exchange benefits and cost sharing would still apply.

Premium assistance. While the bridge plan allows an exchange-eligible family member to be enrolled in a Medicaid plan, CMS recently described an opportunity for Medicaid and CHIP enrollees to be enrolled in a family member's exchange plan (CMS 2013b). As proposed, a state could use existing authority in Medicaid and CHIP for premium assistance to pay the premiums and cost sharing for Medicaid- or CHIP-eligible individuals enrolled in nongroup coverage, including exchange coverage. In describing this option, CMS reiterated that individuals eligible for Medicaid or CHIP cannot receive exchange subsidies and that the premium assistance must be cost effective (CMS 2013b). To be cost effective, the state payments for premium assistance (including administrative expenditures and the costs of providing wraparound benefits) must be comparable to the cost of providing direct Medicaid coverage.

Basic Health Program. Some states are exploring the option of implementing a Basic Health Program, through which states could provide coverage for individuals between 138 and 200 percent FPL. If offered in their state, eligible individuals would be required to enroll in the Basic Health Program in lieu of obtaining subsidized coverage in the exchanges. States would receive 95 percent of the money the federal government would have paid for subsidized exchange coverage.

The purpose of these programs is not only to reduce churning, but also to reduce the likelihood that low-income families would be forced to repay premium tax credits they received should they experience an increase in income or a change in family composition. Prior to the Supreme Court's decision allowing states to forgo the expansion, one study found that 4 percent fewer adults (1.8 million individuals) would churn between Medicaid and exchange coverage if states offered the Basic Health Program option (Hwang et al. 2012). This assumes that the Basic Health Program would be comparable to Medicaid in terms of participating plans and covered benefits, so that the first income-based transition point between markets would be at 200 rather than 138 percent FPL.

In February, CMS announced it plans to issue proposed rules on the Basic Health Program later this year, and that states will not be able to implement a Basic Health Program until 2015 (CMS 2013c).

Twelve-month continuous eligibility. Another avenue by which states may reduce churning is by opting for 12-month continuous eligibility for Medicaid and CHIP enrollees. Under current rules, Medicaid enrollees are generally required to report changes that may affect eligibility between regularly scheduled redeterminations (42 CFR 435.916(c)). Based on these requirements, enrollment in Medicaid can change in any month. Twelve-month continuous eligibility allows states to enroll individuals in Medicaid or CHIP for 12 months, regardless of changes in family income or composition that occur in the interim. Under continuous eligibility, families are not required to report changes in income. There are certain conditions, however, that must still prompt a review of eligibility, such as when a child reaches the age limit.

Twelve-month continuous eligibility is an explicit statutory option for children in Medicaid (§1902(e)(12) of the Act) and is used by 23 states, as shown in Table 2-1 (HHS 2012). Besides using waivers, states are permitted to effectively implement continuous eligibility for adults in Medicaid using current state flexibility to disregard changes in income. However, once MAGI takes effect in 2014, this income-counting flexibility goes away and thus also the flexibility to implement 12-month continuous eligibility for adults in Medicaid without a waiver (CMS 2012c). As with adults in Medicaid, no explicit statutory authority exists for separate CHIP programs to have 12-month continuous eligibility. However, 33 states currently use 12-month continuous eligibility in CHIP (HHS 2012), and CMS is proposing to codify 12-month continuous eligibility for CHIP through regulations so states can be assured of that option continuing in 2014 (CMS 2013b).

Twelve-month continuous eligibility would be of particular importance for individuals with serious and chronic health conditions who receive broader coverage in Medicaid that they might not receive in exchange coverage. Even in subsidized exchange coverage, the costs of needed yet uncovered benefits—or benefits with higher out-of-pocket cost sharing—could be very high for these individuals. Additional costs could also

TABLE 2-1. States Providing Continuous Eligibility to Children

The following states provide 12-month continuous eligibility to children in Medicaid or CHIP.

State	CHIP	Medicaid	State	CHIP	Medicaid
Alabama	Yes	Yes	New Jersey	Yes	Yes
Alaska	Yes	No	New Mexico	Yes	Yes
Arizona	Yes	No	New York	Yes	Yes
California	Yes	Yes	North Carolina	Yes	Yes
Colorado	Yes	No	North Dakota	Yes	Yes
Delaware	Yes	No	Ohio	Yes	Yes
Florida	Yes	No	Oregon	Yes	Yes
Idaho	Yes	Yes	Pennsylvania	Yes	No
Illinois	Yes	Yes	South Carolina	Yes	Yes
Iowa	Yes	Yes	Tennessee	Yes	No
Kansas	Yes	Yes	Texas	Yes	No
Louisiana	Yes	Yes	Utah	Yes	No
Maine	Yes	Yes	Virginia	Yes	Yes
Michigan	Yes	Yes	Washington	Yes	Yes
Mississippi	Yes	Yes	West Virginia	Yes	Yes
Montana	Yes	Yes	Wyoming	Yes	Yes
Nevada	Yes	No			

Note: See source document for some exceptions in Arizona, Pennsylvania, Tennessee, Texas, and Virginia.
Source: CMS 2013d

apply if individuals underestimate their income for purposes of the exchange premium tax credits and then must repay certain amounts at reconciliation during the tax filing process. If individuals are likely to churn between Medicaid and subsidized exchange coverage, it may be beneficial for them, their providers, and the federal and state governments for such individuals to remain in Medicaid for the entire 12-month period.

A study conducted in 2009 found that average monthly Medicaid expenditures were lower the longer children were enrolled in Medicaid (Ku et al. 2009). Continuously enrolled children were found to have more regular preventive care, which improves health and reduces the likelihood of inpatient hospital admissions or costly emergency room visits (Ku et al. 2009). It was also noted that this reduction in costs over time was partly due to the fact that newly enrolled children may have had pent-up demand for services compared to children with consistent coverage.

Commission Recommendation

Recommendation 2.1

In order to ensure that current eligibility options remain available to states in 2014, the Congress should, parallel to the existing Medicaid 12-month continuous eligibility option for children, create a similar statutory option for children enrolled in CHIP and adults enrolled in Medicaid.

Rationale

This recommendation ensures continued flexibility for states to implement 12-month continuous eligibility. States have used this option for years for children in Medicaid and separate CHIP programs. Although CMS is proposing to codify 12-month continuous eligibility in CHIP through regulations (CMS 2013b), explicit statutory authority would further guarantee this state option.

The statutory option to provide 12-month continuous eligibility to children enrolled in Medicaid has functioned under explicit statutory authority since 1997. Although no explicit statutory authority exists for 12-month continuous eligibility in CHIP or for adults in Medicaid, 33 states use existing flexibility to implement it in CHIP (HHS 2012). CMS is proposing to codify 12-month continuous eligibility in CHIP through regulations so states can be assured of that option continuing in 2014 (CMS 2013b).

In making this recommendation, the Commission wants to emphasize the importance of accurate eligibility determinations and meaningful verification of applicants' self-reported information. If states will have the option to keep individuals in Medicaid and CHIP regardless of what are typically modest income changes, then it is critical for both initial determinations and regular redeterminations to reflect the most accurate information available. To accomplish this, it is critical that the executive branch successfully establish the proposed federal data services hub, an electronic service by which applicant information will be verified by authoritative sources—for example, citizenship by the Social Security Administration, immigration status by the Department of Homeland Security, and income data from the IRS (CMS 2012c). While pursuing streamlined, simplified application processes, newly promulgated federal regulations make it appropriately clear that "(n)othing in the regulations in this subpart should be construed as limiting the State's program integrity measures or affecting the State's obligation to ensure that only eligible individuals receive benefits" (CMS 2012c, 42 CFR 435.940).

While no state has implemented 12-month continuous eligibility for adults in Medicaid,[5] states could accomplish it using their current income-counting flexibility, by disregarding income changes within enrollees' 12-month eligibility period. Under MAGI in 2014, however, this flexibility goes away; 12-month continuous eligibility will not be a state plan option for adults in Medicaid beginning in 2014 (CMS 2012c). While states could provide 12-month continuous eligibility through the use of Section 1115 waivers, these waivers must be periodically renewed, meet tests of budget or allotment neutrality, and be subject to evaluation and reporting requirements—all of which would increase states' administrative burdens. Although many policies may be implemented through waivers, the Commission believes that providing sound policy choices through state plan options is preferable to relying on waivers.

As described earlier, 12-month continuous eligibility reduces churning and the negative health effects that may result. Twelve-month continuous eligibility ensures access to care for these enrollees and allows them to maintain their same provider network for the year. This may lead to better health outcomes and help minimize the use of more expensive care, such as costly emergency room visits or avoidable hospital admissions.

While analyses and evaluations of 12-month continuous eligibility are limited, the U.S. Government Accountability Office (GAO) assessed churning within a one-year period under ACA rules in place in 2014, estimating that in states with 12-month continuous eligibility, 3 percent of children with Medicaid or CHIP would experience a change in household income within the year that would affect their eligibility, compared to 30 percent of children in states without 12-month continuous eligibility (GAO 2012a). GAO also noted, "Changes in eligibility caused by income fluctuations could deter children's enrollment in relevant programs if the process for changing enrollment is burdensome for the families and could further complicate other eligibility complexities, such as variation in eligibility within households" (GAO 2012a).

MACPAC has examined continuous eligibility from another perspective, focusing on the average length of children's enrollment in Medicaid in states with 12-month continuous eligibility compared to those without.[6] In states with 12-month continuous eligibility, children were enrolled for an average of 10.01 months per year, compared to 9.66 months for those without—a difference of nearly 4 percent. However, other state-level factors may also affect these numbers, and the effect may be substantially different, depending on the state. For example, when Colorado decided in 2009 to pursue 12-month continuous eligibility for children in Medicaid, the state projected that average length of enrollment would increase by 25 percent—from 8.5 to 10.7 months (Colorado Legislative Council 2009).[7] This large projected change could be driven by the state's relatively low average length of enrollment or other state-specific characteristics.

With respect to adults with income below 200 percent FPL, one study projected that if continuous eligibility were not in place and all states expanded Medicaid, 35 percent of these adults would have income changes that would shift their eligibility from Medicaid to exchange coverage or the reverse in a six-month period in 2014. Within a year, an estimated 50 percent—28 million people—would have income changes requiring a program change (Sommers and Rosenbaum 2011). The authors acknowledge that these estimates do not account for the extent to which people would not actually report such a change.

In a follow-up analysis by the lead author, among adults projected to have an income increase from below to above 138 percent FPL by the end of a 12-month period, 43 percent would still have income below 200 percent FPL, 39 percent would have income between 200 and 400 percent FPL, and 18 percent would have income above 400 percent FPL (Sommers 2013). It is important to note that these estimates make no projections of individuals' coverage—either what they began the year with or, in 2014, what they would obtain after the income change. They simply show the size of income changes for this particular group of individuals. Many of those whose income rises above 400 percent FPL would be younger, better-educated individuals— potentially young adults finishing school or getting new jobs. Notwithstanding any 12-month continuous eligibility, these individuals would no longer be eligible for Medicaid or subsidized exchange coverage if their income were still above 400 percent FPL at their annual redetermination.

Implications

Federal spending. This recommendation would increase federal spending in 2014 by $50 million to $250 million. Over the five-year period of 2014 to 2018, this recommendation would increase federal spending by approximately $1 billion. These are the smallest non-zero categories of spending used by the Congressional Budget Office (CBO) when making budget estimates.

States. This recommendation would continue to provide states the option to offer 12-month continuous eligibility through a state plan option, without needing to obtain waiver approvals and renewals. States taking up this option would face additional costs from enrollees' increased tenure in the program; however, this could be offset to some extent by less spending from medical expenses avoided by consistent coverage. It would also be offset by reduced administrative burden resulting from fewer within-year redeterminations. Nationally, the projected impact on state spending from this recommendation would be less than half of the federal spending.

Enrollees. In states that implement 12-month continuous eligibility, this recommendation would reduce churning by allowing enrollees to maintain their Medicaid or CHIP coverage, thus keeping the same provider network and benefits. This would allow for more consistent access to primary and preventive care. While enrollees would not be required to report income changes, individuals wanting to move between programs because of an income change would still be afforded that opportunity. If implemented, 12-month continuous eligibility would also help ensure parents and their children share the same coverage periods—for example, so that renewal paperwork for the family would come at the same time, regardless of whether some family members are enrolled in Medicaid and others in CHIP. It would also reduce the likelihood that individuals would transition back and forth between Medicaid and subsidized exchange coverage, where they could be liable to repay premium credits if their income projections were not accurate.

Providers. Allowing for 12-month continuous eligibility would reduce administrative burden on providers dealing with individuals' moves between sources of coverage or uninsurance. Consistent coverage can ensure that plans' and providers' efforts to improve the management of enrollees' care are not lost through churning. Because many health care quality measures require individuals to be enrolled in a plan for 12 months, continuous eligibility can improve efforts to measure quality.

Other considerations

The Commission considered a recommendation to require states to institute 12-month continuous eligibility for populations eligible for Medicaid or CHIP based on MAGI. This policy would not have applied to individuals eligible on the basis of being age 65 and over or disabled. Requiring states to provide 12-month continuous eligibility to adults and children enrolled in Medicaid and CHIP would help reduce churning between programs over the course of the year. However, if required of all MAGI-based populations, this policy would increase federal spending by approximately $10 billion over five years. MACPAC plans to conduct additional analyses of 12-month continuous eligibility in the future, to assess its impact on enrollees' duration of coverage and continuity of care, as well as the cost impact on states. Such analyses may provide additional support in the future for a recommendation to implement mandatory 12-month continuous eligibility for certain populations.

Transitional Medical Assistance

Nearly every year, the Congress appropriates funding for a Medicaid provision known as Transitional Medical Assistance (TMA). The most recent extension was included as part of the fiscal cliff legislation enacted at the end of 2012, providing funding for TMA through December 31, 2013 (P.L. 112-240). TMA requires states to provide at least six months, and up to 12 months, of Medicaid coverage to enrollees under Section 1931 (i.e., low-income parents and their children) when the family's income has risen above a state's current eligibility levels. Current eligibility levels for Section 1931 vary widely by state, from 10 percent FPL in Alabama—which is less than $2,000 in annual income for a family of three— to 133 percent FPL or more in several states.

If family income rises above these levels, TMA continues coverage when parents might otherwise become uninsured. TMA is less critical to preventing loss of coverage for children, because other Medicaid and CHIP eligibility pathways exist for children above Section 1931 eligibility levels. In 2014, however, TMA may no longer be necessary to prevent uninsurance in states where the combination of Medicaid, CHIP, and subsidized exchange coverage extends to 400 percent FPL. The remainder of the chapter describes TMA and how its role merits changes beginning in 2014.

Background

Since 1974, TMA has provided extended Medicaid coverage to members of low-income families who would otherwise lose Medicaid and potentially become uninsured because of an increase in hours from employment or increased income from child or spousal support. This coverage is primarily available to parents and their children. The historical purpose of TMA was to provide "protection against loss of Medicaid because of increased earnings" (U.S. House of Representatives 1972). TMA has served as a "key protection offered to families at a critical juncture in their efforts to move from welfare to work" (GAO 2002).

Current TMA enrollment and spending. Information on TMA enrollment and spending is not systematically reported by states. The Secretary was required by a 2009 law to collect information on TMA enrollment and spending through annual reports to the Congress. To date, no such report has been published. According to GAO, "While CMS officials report having received data from some states, officials indicated that they have not enforced the requirement because of competing agency priorities" (GAO 2012b).

In 2012, GAO surveyed states for their TMA enrollment and spending from 2006 through the most current year available. In FY 2011, there were 3.5 million TMA enrollees in 41 states (GAO 2012b). Including states' reported spending following publication of its report, GAO's preliminary findings indicate that TMA spending in FY 2011 totaled $4.1 billion in 36 states.

TMA as originally enacted. Prior to the 1996 enactment of welfare reform, families who were enrolled in the cash welfare program Aid to Families with Dependent Children (AFDC) were automatically eligible for Medicaid. Eligibility levels for AFDC varied by state but were generally only a fraction of the federal poverty level. As a result, relatively small amounts of earnings could disqualify these families from Medicaid. TMA was designed to ensure that these families would retain Medicaid coverage for some time, even with an increase in income that made them ineligible for AFDC. As originally enacted, TMA required states to provide four months of coverage to individuals who had been enrolled in AFDC for at least three of the past six months. This original version of TMA is permanently funded in the Medicaid statute.

Selected major changes in TMA. In 1988, the Congress required states to provide six months of TMA (P.L. 100-485). States were also required to provide an additional six months of TMA—for a total of 12 months—for families below 185 percent FPL who provided quarterly reports of their earnings and work-related child care expenses in the 4th, 7th, and 10th months of TMA enrollment. Unlike most Medicaid policies, this TMA change was not permanently funded; funding was provided for 10 years, through September 30, 1998.

The 1988 legislation also provided states with a "wrap-around option" (§1925(a)(4)(B) of the Act). This permits the state to pay for the premiums and cost sharing for ESI that may be available to a person eligible for Medicaid through TMA. Indeed, the state may require such individuals to enroll in that employment-based coverage as a condition of receiving TMA. In GAO's recent survey, 23 states reported using this premium assistance option for some of their TMA enrollees (GAO 2012b).

The 1996 welfare reform law replaced AFDC with Temporary Assistance for Needy Families (TANF) and broke the automatic eligibility link between welfare and Medicaid. In its place, Section 1931 was added to Medicaid so that individuals who would have been eligible based on the AFDC rules in place on July 16, 1996, would be eligible for Medicaid. Since then, TMA has been available to individuals losing eligibility through Section 1931 rather than the defunct AFDC program.

Current eligibility levels for parents vary widely by state, from 10 percent FPL in Alabama to 133 percent FPL or more in several states. Coverage under Section 1931 and TMA are virtually the only current state plan options for non-disabled, low-income parents. Since the enactment of TMA, however, additional pathways for children have been added such that Medicaid and CHIP coverage is at or above 200 percent FPL in the vast majority of states. Thus, TMA has a much smaller role in preventing uninsurance for children than it does for their parents.

The American Recovery and Reinvestment Act of 2009 (ARRA, P.L. 111-5) made numerous changes to TMA. Consistent with a GAO recommendation (GAO 1999), ARRA gave states the option to waive the requirements unique to TMA enrollees in the second six-month period (i.e., requirements to report earnings and child care and to remain below 185 percent FPL)—sometimes referred to as the 12-month option. ARRA also provided states with the option to waive the requirement that individuals be enrolled in Medicaid for three out of the past six months in order to qualify for TMA. Several states have implemented these state plan options (CMS 2012d):

- Alaska, Colorado, Maryland, Ohio, and Oregon permit the second six-month period of TMA to be treated like the first, without additional reporting requirements; and

- Oregon also permits individuals to be eligible for TMA after only one month of Section 1931 enrollment, rather than three out of the last six months.

Prior to these state plan options, some states achieved these policy changes through waivers (Grady 2008).

For the past several years, funding for current TMA has continued through short-term extensions. For example, one law extended its funding from December 31, 2011, to February 29, 2012, and another from February 29 to December 31, 2012. Most recently, P.L. 112-240 extended TMA funding through December 31, 2013.

As these extensions have been perennial issues for the Congress, they have also been perennial issues for states faced with the uncertainty of whether current TMA would continue or would revert to the permanently funded four-month TMA. This uncertainty concerning TMA's future has also affected federal guidance. Recent proposed regulations only addressed four-month TMA, not the current TMA that has been in effect for years (CMS 2013b).

TMA in 2014

Beginning in 2014, the primary role of TMA to prevent uninsurance may no longer be applicable in states where parents could be eligible for Medicaid up to 138 percent FPL and for subsidized exchange coverage up to 400 percent FPL. Nevertheless, CMS has noted that the ACA did not remove any of the current requirements of TMA (CMS 2012c, CMS 2012e). Because of the Supreme Court's decision that effectively allows states to opt out of the Medicaid expansion, TMA will still be relevant in those states to prevent uninsurance.

States that do not expand Medicaid. In states that do not expand Medicaid in 2014, an eligibility gap will likely exist between Section 1931 coverage and subsidized exchange coverage, as previously discussed and illustrated in Figure 2-1. For these states, TMA would help bridge that gap for Medicaid enrollees whose income increases and should therefore be preserved, consistent with TMA's intent of preventing uninsurance.

States that expand Medicaid. In states that expand Medicaid to the new adult group such that there is no eligibility gap with subsidized exchange coverage, TMA will no longer be as necessary to prevent uninsurance. Compared to the relatively low Section 1931 eligibility rates for parents, Medicaid coverage in these states will be available to parents (and childless adults) up to at least 138 percent FPL and subsidized exchange coverage up to 400 percent FPL. Under current law, however, TMA eligibility would override eligibility for coverage through the new adult group or through exchanges. For example, individuals eligible for TMA will be ineligible for subsidized exchange coverage (§36B(c)(2)(B) of the Internal Revenue Code, as added by §1401(a) of the ACA). While extending TMA will provide these individuals with Medicaid's more generous benefits and cost-sharing protections regardless of their income, it will be at additional state cost, since TMA requires state matching payments while subsidized exchange coverage does not.

Commission Recommendation

Recommendation 2.2

The Congress should permanently fund current Transitional Medical Assistance (TMA) (required for six months, with state option for 12 months), while allowing states to opt out of TMA if they expand to the new adult group added under the Patient Protection and Affordable Care Act.

Rationale

For years, TMA has reduced churning and prevented uninsurance by providing low-income families with six months or more of Medicaid when their income rises above Section 1931 levels. In states that expand Medicaid to the new adult group such that there is no eligibility gap with subsidized exchange coverage, TMA may no longer be as necessary to prevent uninsurance. Its continuation could create unnecessary confusion and administrative burden for enrollees and state governments. Its elimination in states expanding to the new adult group would reduce their Medicaid spending and simplify eligibility by removing the federal statutory requirement to provide TMA.

Although subsidized exchange coverage will exist in every state, the Medicaid expansions to the new adult group may not. In those states where an eligibility gap will exist between Medicaid and subsidized exchange coverage, TMA in its current form should continue for those parents who would otherwise become uninsured. This change should be made permanent so that states do not have to perennially question whether current TMA will be available.

Implications

Federal spending. This recommendation would increase federal spending in 2014 by $50 million to $250 million. Over the five-year period of 2014 to 2018, this recommendation would decrease federal spending by less than $1 billion.

The two components of the recommendation have offsetting effects on federal spending. Extending current TMA provides small federal savings. Federal savings occur because extending TMA puts people in Medicaid who would otherwise have gone to subsidized exchange coverage, which is projected to be more expensive to the federal government than Medicaid (CBO 2012). The other component of the recommendation would have some individuals go into exchange coverage rather than remain in TMA, which increases federal spending by a relatively small amount. Combining these two components, the recommendation's one-year and five-year cost estimates are in the smallest non-zero categories used by the CBO. In both cases, the estimates are in the lower end of the range.

States. If current TMA were allowed to expire, states would have to change their eligibility systems to adapt to the permanently funded four months of TMA. In states that implement the expansion to the new adult group, TMA could create unnecessary confusion and administrative burden for state governments. For example, if at a redetermination enrollees are determined eligible for subsidized exchange coverage rather than Section 1931 Medicaid, the extension of TMA would require those individuals to remain in Medicaid for at least another six months, after which they would undergo another redetermination.

In states that do not implement the expansion to the new adult group, the extension of TMA would essentially continue the status quo. However, because the CBO's baseline assumption is that TMA reverts to its original four-month duration on January 1, 2014, its extension is treated as a state cost of about $300 million in 2014 and $3 billion over five years. Nevertheless, as with past TMA extensions, many states are likely planning on TMA continuing and may not consider this new spending. For states implementing the expansion and opting out of TMA, state spending would be reduced by approximately $100 million in 2014 and $200 million over five years.

Enrollees. In states that do not implement the expansion, this recommendation would ensure TMA exists to provide six months or more of Medicaid—coverage that could prevent uninsurance. In states implementing the expansion, TMA could create unnecessary confusion and administrative burden as TMA provides an additional six months or more of Section 1931 coverage. On the other hand, in the absence of TMA, individuals moving from Medicaid into exchange coverage, even when subsidized, will face higher out-of-pocket cost sharing than required in Medicaid. This is also true of individuals whose income is above 138 percent FPL but who do not qualify for exchange subsidies because their ESI is considered affordable under the ACA.

Providers. Effects on providers would be largest where TMA's extension prevents uninsurance. Otherwise, effects on providers should be minimal.

Endnotes

1 The Court's ruling held that "the Medicaid expansion violates the Constitution by threatening States with the loss of their existing Medicaid funding if they decline to comply with the expansion" (*NFIB v. Sebelius*, p. 4). Section 1904 of the Social Security Act—a provision of Medicaid law that has been in existence unaltered since Medicaid's enactment in 1965—says that if a state Medicaid program is out of compliance with federal requirements, the Secretary has the authority to withhold federal funding for the part that is out of compliance or from the state's entire Medicaid program. In *NFIB v. Sebelius*, the Court determined that the Secretary cannot withhold all Medicaid funds from states not implementing the expansion. The Court did so by reasoning that the expansion is, in fact, a new program separate from current Medicaid because the new adult group (1) is a new eligibility group inconsistent with Medicaid's historical eligibility categories, (2) is reimbursed at a federal matching rate inconsistent with Medicaid's typical matching rate, and (3) will receive a mandated benefit package unique from any other required for an eligibility group at the federal level (*NFIB v. Sebelius*, pp. 53–54).

2 Several other states cover childless adults by using Section 1115 waivers (KFF 2012).

3 Even for applicants who file tax returns, their Medicaid eligibility is to be determined based on their current income (§1902(e)(14)(H) of the Act, 42 CFR 603(h)). Thus, for Medicaid purposes, the use of information from previous tax returns will likely be limited to verifying that it is reasonably compatible with current income (42 CFR 952).

4 Nineteen states use a separate CHIP program to cover 6- to 18-year-olds between 100 and 133 percent FPL: Alabama, Arizona, California, Colorado, Delaware, Florida, Georgia, Kansas, Mississippi, Nevada, North Carolina, North Dakota, Oregon, Pennsylvania, Tennessee, Texas, Utah, West Virginia, and Wyoming. In 2012, New Hampshire and New York modified their CHIP programs to place these children in a Medicaid expansion.

5 New York has approval under its Section 1115 waiver to provide 12-month continuous eligibility to parents (CMS 2012f) but has not yet implemented this provision (KFF 2013).

6 This analysis used data from the FY 2009 Medicaid Statistical Information System annual person summary data from CMS. Only states with 12-month (rather than 6-month) renewal periods were included. States' Medicaid renewal periods and continuous eligibility policies were from the Kaiser Family Foundation (KFF 2009).

7 Colorado has not yet implemented 12-month continuous eligibility for children in Medicaid.

References

Bindman, A.B., A. Chattopadhyay, and G.M. Auerback. 2008. Interruptions in Medicaid coverage and risk for hospitalization for ambulatory care-sensitive conditions. *Annuals of Internal Medicine* 149, no. 12: 854–860.

Buettgens, M., A. Nichols, and S. Dorn. 2012. *Churning under the ACA and state policy options for mitigation.* Washington, DC: Urban Institute. http://www.urban.org/UploadedPDF/412587-Churning-Under-the-ACA-and-State-Policy-Options-for-Mitigation.pdf.

Centers for Medicare & Medicaid Services (CMS), U.S. Department of Health and Human Services. 2013a. Patient Protection and Affordable Care Act; Exchange functions: Eligibility for exemptions; Miscellaneous minimum essential coverage provisions. Proposed rule. *Federal Register* 78, no. 22 (February 1): 7348–7371.

Centers for Medicare & Medicaid Services (CMS), U.S. Department of Health and Human Services. 2013b. Medicaid, Children's Health Insurance Programs, and Exchanges: Essential health benefits in alternative benefit plans; eligibility notices; fair hearing and appeal processes for Medicaid and exchange eligibility appeals and other provisions related to eligibility and enrollment for exchanges, Medicaid and CHIP, and Medicaid premiums and cost sharing. Proposed rule. *Federal Register* 78, no. 14 (January 22): 4594–4724.

Centers for Medicare & Medicaid Services (CMS), U.S. Department of Health and Human Services. 2013c. *Questions and answers: Medicaid and the Affordable Care Act.* http://www.medicaid.gov/State-Resource-Center/Frequently-Asked-Questions/Downloads/ACA-FAQ-BHP.pdf.

Centers for Medicare & Medicaid Services (CMS), U.S. Department of Health and Human Services. 2013d. Continuous eligibility for Medicaid and CHIP coverage. http://www.insurekidsnow.gov/professionals/eligibility/continuous.html.

Centers for Medicare & Medicaid Services (CMS), U.S. Department of Health and Human Services. 2012a. *Frequently asked questions on exchanges, market reforms and Medicaid.* http://medicaid.gov/State-Resource-Center/Frequently-Asked-Questions/Downloads/Governor-FAQs-12-10-12.pdf.

Centers for Medicare & Medicaid Services (CMS), U.S. Department of Health and Human Services. 2012b. Letter from Marilyn Tavenner to Daniel R. Levinson regarding "Office of Inspector General (OIG) draft report: Most states anticipate implementing streamlined eligibility and enrollment by 2014 (OEI-07-10-00530)." December 20, 2012. https://oig.hhs.gov/oei/reports/oei-07-10-00530.pdf.

Centers for Medicare & Medicaid Services (CMS), U.S. Department of Health and Human Services. 2012c. Medicaid program; Eligibility changes under the Affordable Care Act of 2010. Final rule. *Federal Register* 77, no. 57 (March 23): 17143–17217. http://www.gpo.gov/fdsys/pkg/FR-2012-03-23/html/2012-6560.htm.

Centers for Medicare & Medicaid Services (CMS), U.S. Department of Health and Human Services. 2012d. *Medicaid state plan amendments.* http://www.medicaid.gov/State-Resource-Center/Medicaid-State-Plan-Amendments/Medicaid-State-Plan-Amendments.html.

Centers for Medicare & Medicaid Services (CMS), U.S. Department of Health and Human Services. 2012e. *Medicaid/CHIP Affordable Care Act implementation: Answers to frequently asked questions—Eligibility policy.* http://www.medicaid.gov/State-Resource-Center/Frequently-Asked-Questions/Downloads/Eligibility-Policy-FAQs.pdf.

Centers for Medicare & Medicaid Services (CMS), U.S. Department of Health and Human Services. 2012f. *Centers for Medicare & Medicaid Services special terms and conditions: Federal-state health reform partnership Medicaid Section 1115 demonstration.* http://www.medicaid.gov/Medicaid-CHIP-Program-Information/By-Topics/Waivers/1115/downloads/ny/ny-f-shrp-ca.pdf.

Centers for Medicare & Medicaid Services (CMS), U.S. Department of Health and Human Services. 2011a. Letter from Cindy Mann to State Medicaid Directors, regarding "Maintenance of effort." February 25, 2011. http://downloads.cms.gov/cmsgov/archived-downloads/SMDL/downloads/SMD11001.pdf.

Centers for Medicare & Medicaid Services (CMS), U.S. Department of Health and Human Services. 2011b. Medicaid program; Federal funding for Medicaid eligibility determination and enrollment activities. Final rule. *Federal Register* 76, no. 75 (April 19): 21950–21975.

Colorado Legislative Council, State of Colorado. 2009. *Final fiscal note,* HB09-1293. http://www.leg.state.co.us/clics/clics2009a/csl.nsf/billcontainers/D71C48DD229F80CD872575540079F3A0/$FILE/HB1293_f1.pdf.

Congressional Budget Office (CBO). 2013a. *CBO's February 2013 estimate of the effects of the Affordable Care Act on health insurance coverage.* Washington, DC: CBO. http://www.cbo.gov/sites/default/files/cbofiles/attachments/43900_ACAInsuranceCoverageEffects.pdf.

Congressional Budget Office (CBO). 2013b. *The budget and economic outlook: Fiscal years 2013 to 2023.* Washington, DC: CBO. http://www.cbo.gov/sites/default/files/cbofiles/attachments/43907-BudgetOutlook.pdf.

Congressional Budget Office (CBO). 2012. *Estimates for the insurance coverage provisions of the Affordable Care Act updated for the recent Supreme Court decision.* Washington, DC: CBO. http://www.cbo.gov/sites/default/files/cbofiles/attachments/43472-07-24-2012-CoverageEstimates.pdf.

Czajka, J.L. 2012. *Movement of children between Medicaid and CHIP, 2005–2007.* MAX Medicaid policy brief no. 4. Princeton, NJ: Mathematica Policy Research, Inc. http://www.cms.gov/Research-Statistics-Data-and-Systems/Computer-Data-and-Systems/MedicaidDataSourcesGenInfo/Downloads/Medicaid_and_CHIP_Transitions.pdf.

Czajka, J.L., and J. Mabli. 2009. *Analysis of transition events in health insurance coverage: Final report.* Washington, DC: Mathematica Policy Research, Inc. http://aspe.hhs.gov/health/reports/09/CoverageTransitions/index.shtml.

Fairbrother, G., and J. Schuchter. 2008. *Stability and churning in Medi-Cal and healthy families.* Los Angeles, CA: The California Endowment. http://www.cincinnatichildrens.org/assets/0/78/1067/1395/1833/1835/9811/9813/9819/48b3047a-79ac-4e52-9ed8-b7824db1cec3.pdf.

Finocchio, L. 2012. Medi-Cal: An overview of the managed care delivery system. Presentation before the National Academy for State Health Policy, October 16, 2012, Baltimore, MD.

Grady, A. 2008. *Transitional Medical Assistance (TMA) under Medicaid.* Report no. RL31698. Washington, DC: Congressional Research Service. http://assets.opencrs.com/rpts/RL31698_20040630.pdf.

Hall, A.G., J.S. Harman, and J. Zhang. 2008. Lapses in Medicaid coverage: Impact on cost and utilization among individuals with diabetes enrolled in Medicaid. *Medical Care* 46, no. 12: 1219–1225.

Harman, J.S., A.G. Hall, and J. Zhang. 2007. Changes in health care use and costs after a break in Medicaid coverage among persons with depression. *Psychiatric Services* 58, no. 1: 49–54.

Hwang, A., S. Rosenbaum, and B.D. Sommers. 2012. Creation of state basic health programs would lead to 4 percent fewer people churning between Medicaid and exchanges. *Health Affairs* 31, no. 6: 1314–1320.

Ingram, C., S. McMahon, and V. Guerra. 2012. *Creating seamless coverage transitions between Medicaid and the exchanges.* Issue brief. Princeton, NJ: Center for Health Care Strategies, Inc. http://www.statenetwork.org/resource/creating-seamless-coverage-transitions-between-medicaid-and-the-exchanges/.

Kaiser Family Foundation (KFF). 2013. *Getting into gear for 2014: Findings from a 50-state survey of eligibility, enrollment, renewal, and cost-sharing policies in Medicaid and CHIP, 2012–2013.* Washington, DC: Kaiser Commission on Medicaid and the Uninsured. http://www.kff.org/medicaid/upload/8401.pdf.

Kaiser Family Foundation (KFF). 2012. *Where are states today? Medicaid and CHIP eligibility levels for children and non-disabled adults.* Washington, DC: Kaiser Commission on Medicaid and the Uninsured. http://www.kff.org/medicaid/upload/7993-02.pdf.

Kaiser Family Foundation (KFF). 2010. *Medicaid: A primer.* Washington, DC: Kaiser Commission on Medicaid and the Uninsured. http://www.kff.org/medicaid/upload/7334-04.pdf.

Kaiser Family Foundation (KFF). 2009. *Challenges of providing health coverage for children and parents in a recession: A 50-state update on eligibility rules, enrollment and renewal procedures, and cost-sharing practices in Medicaid and SCHIP in 2009.* Washington, DC: Kaiser Commission on Medicaid and the Uninsured. http://www.kff.org/medicaid/upload/7855.pdf.

Ku, L., P. MacTaggart, and F. Pervez, et al. 2009. *Improving Medicaid's continuity of coverage and quality of care.* Washington, DC: Association for Community Affiliated Plans. http://sphhs.gwu.edu/departments/healthpolicy/dhp_publications/pub_uploads/dhpPublication_66898AB4-5056-9D20-3D5FC0235271FE99.pdf.

Leitz, S. 2013. Interactions between Medicaid, CHIP, and the exchanges: Plan participation. Presentation before the Medicaid and CHIP Payment and Access Commission, January 15, 2013, Washington, DC. http://www.macpac.gov/home/meetings.

Lovelace, J. 2013. Interactions between Medicaid, CHIP, and the exchanges: Plan participation. Presentation before the Medicaid and CHIP Payment and Access Commission, January 15, 2013, Washington, DC. http://www.macpac.gov/home/meetings.

National Federation of Independent Business, et al. v. Kathleen Sebelius, Secretary of Health and Human Services, et al., 567 U.S. ___ (U.S. Supreme Court 2012).

Sommers, B. 2013. Analysis of 2008 SIPP data for MACPAC. Unpublished.

Sommers, B. 2009. Loss of health insurance among non-elderly adults in Medicaid. *Journal of General Internal Medicine* 24, no. 1: 1–7.

Sommers, B., and S. Rosenbaum. 2011. Issues in health reform: How changes in eligibility may move millions back and forth between Medicaid and insurance exchanges. *Health Affairs* 30, no. 2: 228–236.

Summer, L., and C. Mann. 2006. *Instability of public health insurance coverage for children and their families: Causes, consequences, and remedies.* Washington, DC: Commonwealth Fund. http://www.commonwealthfund.org/usr_doc/Summer_instabilitypubhltinschildren_935.pdf.

Tennessee Insurance Exchange Planning Initiative (IEPI), State of Tennessee. 2011. *Bridge option: One family, one card across time.* http://www.tn.gov/nationalhealthreform/forms/onefamily.pdf.

U.S. Department of Health and Human Services (HHS). 2012. *Continuous eligibility for Medicaid and CHIP coverage.* Washington, DC: HHS. http://www.insurekidsnow.gov/professionals/eligibility/continuous.html.

U.S. Government Accountability Office (GAO). 2012a. *Children's health insurance: Opportunities exist for improved access to affordable insurance.* Report no. GAO-12-648. Washington, DC: GAO. http://www.gao.gov/assets/600/591797.pdf.

U.S. Government Accountability Office (GAO). 2012b. *Medicaid: Enrollment and expenditures for qualified individual and transitional medical assistance programs.* Report no. GAO-13-177R. Washington, DC: GAO. http://www.gao.gov/assets/660/650816.pdf.

U.S. General Accounting Office (GAO). 2002. *Medicaid: Transitional coverage can help families move from welfare to work.* Report no. GAO-02-679T. Washington, DC: GAO. http://www.gao.gov/assets/110/109281.pdf.

U.S. General Accounting Office (GAO). 1999. *Amid declines, state efforts to ensure coverage after welfare reform vary.* Report no. HEHS-99-163. Washington, DC: GAO. http://www.gao.gov/assets/230/228144.pdf.

U.S. House of Representatives. 1972. Summary of H.R. 1, the Social Security Amendments of 1972 as approved by the conferees. Washington, DC. *Congressional Record,* October 17, 1972, p. 36919.

CHAPTER 3

The Roles of Medicare and Medicaid for a Diverse Dual-Eligible Population

Key Points

The Roles of Medicare and Medicaid for a Diverse Dual-Eligible Population

- Persons dually eligible for Medicare and Medicaid are a diverse population, with widely varying care needs and patterns of Medicare and Medicaid service use and spending.

- Among all-year, full-benefit dual eligibles in 2007, 59 percent used no Medicaid long-term services and supports (LTSS) and 41 percent used some LTSS, including 19 percent who used institutional services, 10 percent who used Medicaid home and community-based waiver services as an alternative to institutionalization, and 11 percent who used Medicaid state-plan LTSS only.

- Average annual Medicare and Medicaid spending varied widely across these four groups, from $70,000 for people who used institutional services in Medicaid to about $15,000 for people who did not use any LTSS.

- Full-benefit dual eligibles who did not use LTSS relied almost exclusively on Medicare. They accounted for 59 percent of all-year, full-benefit dual-eligible enrollees but just 11 percent of Medicaid spending on those dual eligibles. They accounted for 30 percent of Medicare spending on the all-year, full-benefit dual-eligible population, however.

- In contrast, people who needed an institutional level of care (who used Medicaid institutional LTSS or waiver services) relied much more heavily on Medicaid and accounted for the majority of Medicaid spending on all-year, full-benefit dual eligibles (78 percent).

- A variety of approaches will be needed to target solutions to the problems faced by these distinct subgroups with diverse needs, service use, and spending in Medicare and Medicaid.

CHAPTER 3

The Roles of Medicare and Medicaid for a Diverse Dual-Eligible Population

Individuals who are dually eligible are low-income seniors and persons with disabilities who are enrolled in both Medicare and Medicaid. In 2011, there were 10.2 million dual eligibles, including 7.5 million people with Medicare who qualified for full Medicaid benefits (full-benefit dual eligibles) and 2.7 million partial-benefit dual eligibles for whom Medicaid provided more limited financial assistance in paying for Medicare premiums or cost sharing (CMS 2013).

The two programs serve distinct roles and together address the needs of a diverse population. For all dual eligibles, Medicare is the primary source of health insurance, covering physician services, inpatient and outpatient hospital care, post-acute care, and prescription drugs. Medicaid fills in gaps in Medicare's coverage, providing financial assistance with Medicare costs for poor and near-poor Medicare beneficiaries, as well as access to services not covered by Medicare, including a wide range of long-term services and supports (LTSS), behavioral health services, vision and dental care, and other wraparound services.

Persons dually eligible for Medicare and Medicaid have been of particular interest to policymakers because they account for a relatively small share of enrollees in each program, but for a disproportionately large share of the expenditures in each. There is also concern that no single entity is responsible for dual eligibles because their care is financed by two separate programs. At times, the two programs appear to work at cross purposes to each other, as there may be incentives for cost shifting that compromise quality of care and raise overall costs. For example, Medicaid costs can be shifted to Medicare when nursing home residents whose care is covered by Medicaid are hospitalized for conditions that could have been managed in the nursing home. Similarly, if post-acute transitions are not properly managed, people who might otherwise have been successfully transitioned from the hospital to the community may instead end up as long-term nursing home residents, increasing costs for Medicaid.

Finally, researchers and health professionals who provide services to dual eligibles point to missed opportunities to provide appropriate, person-centered services that could help prevent predictable consequences of chronic illness and disability, improve health and well-being, and lower overall health care costs (Master 2012, Master and Eng 2001, Whitelaw and Warden 1999). The health care service delivery system does not always meet the needs of people with serious chronic conditions or disabilities who require ongoing care across multiple providers and settings. Too often, health care services for people with chronic illness and disability are fragmented and episodic. These gaps may be problematic for dual eligibles with extensive care needs—and especially for those with limited family and social supports.

Concerns about the quality of care provided to dual eligibles—and about the costs of their care—have prompted growing attention to policy reforms that may improve quality and potentially lower total Medicare and Medicaid costs. The Patient Protection and Affordable Care Act (ACA, P.L. 111–148, as amended) included a number of provisions designed to address policy issues relevant to dual eligibles, establishing a Federal Coordinated Health Care Office (Medicare-Medicaid Coordination Office) and a Center for Medicare and Medicaid Innovation, both of which are involved in efforts to improve care for dual eligibles (CMS 2011).

Dual eligibles, however, are a diverse group, including people who are young and old, people who are relatively healthy as well as those who are gravely ill, and people who have no disabling or chronic conditions as well as those with significant disabilities who require nearly constant supervision. The diversity of the population is reflected in its widely varying use of services and spending in Medicare and Medicaid, with some people having very high spending, mostly for Medicaid LTSS, and others who are relatively healthy and who have low spending that is covered mostly by Medicare. Variation in needs and patterns of service use suggest that dual-eligible subpopulations likely face different challenges in accessing high-quality care. Consequently, different policy approaches will be needed to address the specific challenges faced by diverse subgroups.

To shed light on how the diversity of the dually eligible population may affect the design of policy solutions, we analyzed service use and spending for Medicare and Medicaid services for four distinct groups. Because LTSS use accounts for the majority of Medicaid spending for dual eligibles, our analysis focuses on four groups defined by their use of LTSS. We focus in this chapter on individuals who are fully eligible for both Medicare and Medicaid. Chapter 4 provides more information on the Medicare Savings Programs (MSPs), which assist low-income Medicare beneficiaries with their premiums and cost sharing but do not provide them with full Medicaid benefits.

This chapter begins with a brief overview of the roles of the Medicare and Medicaid programs for dual eligibles, including the benefits financed under each program and how these benefits address the needs of dually eligible individuals. Next, it provides a profile of dual eligibles' service use and spending across the two programs, focusing on the variation in their health care and supportive service needs—with a particular focus on LTSS in Medicaid. The Commission sees this analysis as an important first step in considering how current policy should be changed, both to address concerns about quality and costs and to ensure that the two programs are aligned to best meet the needs of the beneficiaries they serve.

Characteristics of Dual Eligibles

The majority of dually eligible individuals are adults age 65 and older who qualify for Medicare on the basis of their entitlement to a Social Security retirement benefit; other dual eligibles are under age 65 and are enrolled in Medicare as a result of a serious disability.[1] In 2007, 58 percent of dual eligibles were age 65 and older, and 42 percent were under age 65 (Figure 3-1). A far lower percentage of non-dually eligible beneficiaries in Medicare, just 12 percent in 2007, were under age 65 (Coughlin et al. 2012).

Dual eligibles who are 65 and over are often enrolled in Medicare first and then become eligible for Medicaid, typically when they need LTSS, such as care in a nursing home. Other dual eligibles are first enrolled in Medicaid and then become eligible for Medicare when they reach the end of the two-year waiting period for Social Security Disability Insurance (SSDI) benefits, for example.

Because Medicaid's assistance is means-tested, nearly all dually eligible individuals are poor or have very low income and limited financial assets. More than half of all dual eligibles in 2007 (53.4 percent) had an annual income below $10,000 compared to just 8.3 percent of other Medicare beneficiaries (Coughlin et al. 2012).

Medicare's Role for Dual Eligibles

For all dual eligibles, Medicare serves as the primary payer for health care services. Medicare provides coverage for medically necessary physician services and outpatient services (through Part B), inpatient hospital services, rehabilitative therapies, home health care, hospice care, and skilled nursing facility (SNF) care (through Part A), as well as coverage for prescription drugs (through Part D). In 2007, Medicare spending per all-year, full-benefit dual eligible averaged about $16,000. Just over half of their average spending was for inpatient hospital services and prescription drugs; roughly a quarter was for physician and outpatient services (Figure 3-2).

Why do people with Medicare need Medicaid?

Medicare has various exclusions and limitations that matter for persons who are frail or have disabilities. Medicare's traditional health insurance benefit package does not meet the needs of many frail adults age 65 and older or of non-aged persons with disabilities, including those with intellectual and developmental disabilities, physical disabilities like quadriplegia, or disabling conditions like cerebral palsy, multiple sclerosis, mental illnesses such as schizophrenia, and severe emotional conditions. For example, Medicare does

FIGURE 3-1. Dual Eligibles, by Age, 2007

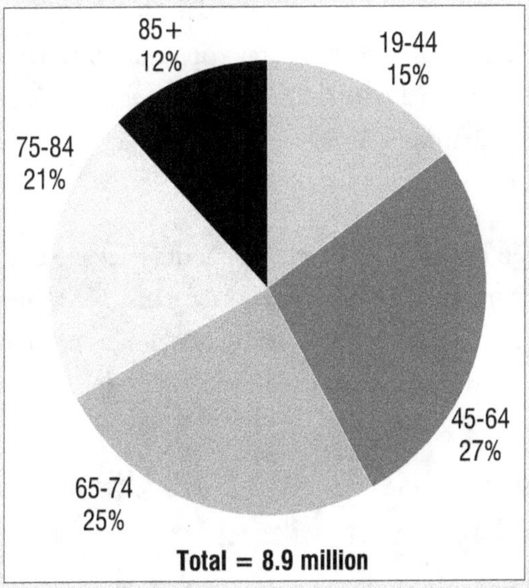

- 85+: 12%
- 19-44: 15%
- 45-64: 27%
- 65-74: 25%
- 75-84: 21%

Total = 8.9 million

Note: Children under age 19 are 0.03% of the dually eligible population.
Source: Mathematica Policy Research analysis of Medicare and Medicaid data for MACPAC

FIGURE 3-2. Average Medicare Spending per All-Year, Full-Benefit Dually Eligible Beneficiary, by Type of Service, 2007

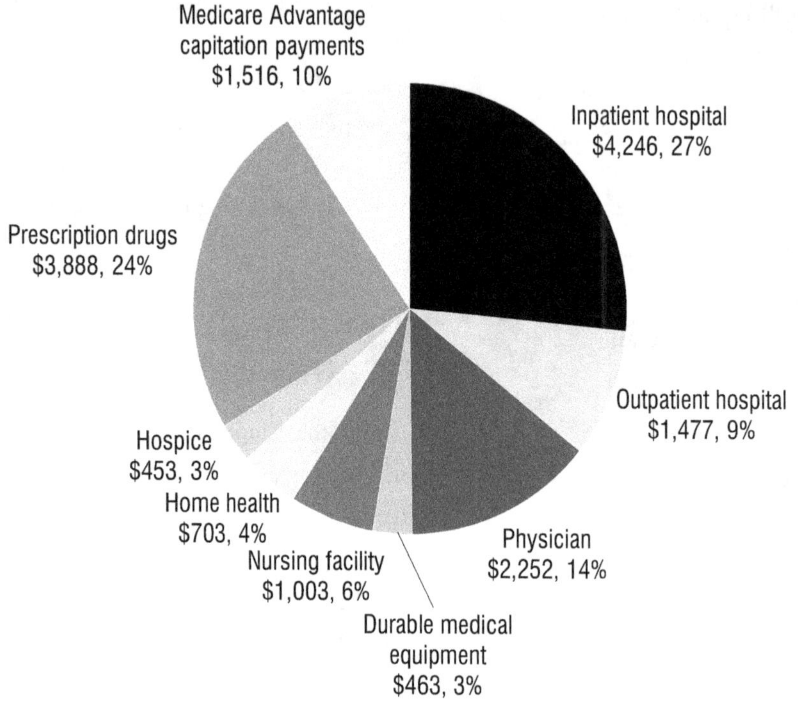

- Medicare Advantage capitation payments $1,516, 10%
- Inpatient hospital $4,246, 27%
- Outpatient hospital $1,477, 9%
- Physician $2,252, 14%
- Durable medical equipment $463, 3%
- Nursing facility $1,003, 6%
- Home health $703, 4%
- Hospice $453, 3%
- Prescription drugs $3,888, 24%

Average Medicare spending per all-year, full-benefit dually eligible beneficiary = $16,001

Note: Physician spending also includes some other Part B spending, including lab and x-ray.
Source: Mathematica Policy Research analysis of Medicare and Medicaid data for MACPAC

not cover supportive services, extended home care for people who are frail, long-term custodial nursing home care, hearing aids, vision care, dental care, or non-emergency transportation services. Medicare covers nursing home services only in skilled facilities and only for beneficiaries who have had a minimum three-day prior hospital stay and who have skilled care needs. Medicare covers home health care only for individuals who need skilled care on a part-time or intermittent basis and who are homebound.

Medicare also requires significant contributions from beneficiaries in the form of premiums, coinsurance, and deductibles. For example, in 2013 Medicare beneficiaries pay a deductible of $1,184 for a hospital stay (of under 60 days) and additional cost sharing for longer inpatient stays. Chapter 4 discusses Medicare's cost-sharing requirements in more detail.

Given limits to Medicare's benefits package and substantial cost-sharing requirements, Medicaid plays an important role for dual eligibles in filling gaps and supplementing needed benefits.

How do people with Medicare qualify for Medicaid?

People with Medicare come into Medicaid through different eligibility pathways. Some people with Medicare come into Medicaid via the Medicare Savings Programs (MSPs). Through the MSPs, Medicaid provides assistance with Medicare premiums and cost sharing to Medicare beneficiaries with very limited income and financial resources—covering out-of-pocket costs that can be unaffordable for the lowest-income people with Medicare. The 2.7 million individuals enrolled only in these programs—who are not otherwise eligible for Medicaid—are considered partial-benefit dual eligibles and are not included in the analysis in this chapter. Chapter 4 provides more information on the MSPs.

Other dually eligible individuals qualify for Medicaid through eligibility pathways that are available to people regardless of their eligibility for Medicare and that provide access to full Medicaid benefits. Some of these pathways are available only to people who are frail or who have serious disabling conditions that meet the standards for nursing home or other long-term institutional care (such as intermediate care facilities for persons with intellectual disabilities (ICFs/ID)).

For these dually eligible individuals, Medicaid covers items and services that are not covered by Medicare, most importantly LTSS, but also mental health and behavioral health therapy and services (when they are not covered by Medicare), transportation services, and case management services, for example. Most, but not all, of these full-benefit dual eligibles also receive assistance from Medicaid with Medicare premiums and cost sharing.

The majority of dual eligibles (7.5 million of the 10.2 million dual eligibles in 2011) have full Medicaid coverage (Figure 3-3). There are four major categories of full-benefit dual eligibles:

People receiving Supplemental Security Income (SSI) cash payments. SSI is available to persons 65 and over, children, and adults with disabilities who are younger than 65 and who have income below poverty (below 75 percent of the federal poverty level) and very limited assets ($2,000 for an individual, $3,000 for a married couple). In most states (39 states and the District of Columbia), people who receive SSI are automatically enrolled in Medicaid. However, 11 states (so-called "209(b)" states) use financial eligibility criteria that are more restrictive than those that apply in the federal SSI program.[2] These states must offer a medically needy pathway to eligibility for very low-income people with medical or supportive service needs.

Poverty-related eligibility. States have the option of providing Medicaid coverage to people who receive a state supplementation payment in addition to SSI. States also have the option to extend Medicaid eligibility to people otherwise eligible for SSI—whose income exceeds the SSI limit, but who have annual income below the federal poverty level. In 2012, 22 states and the

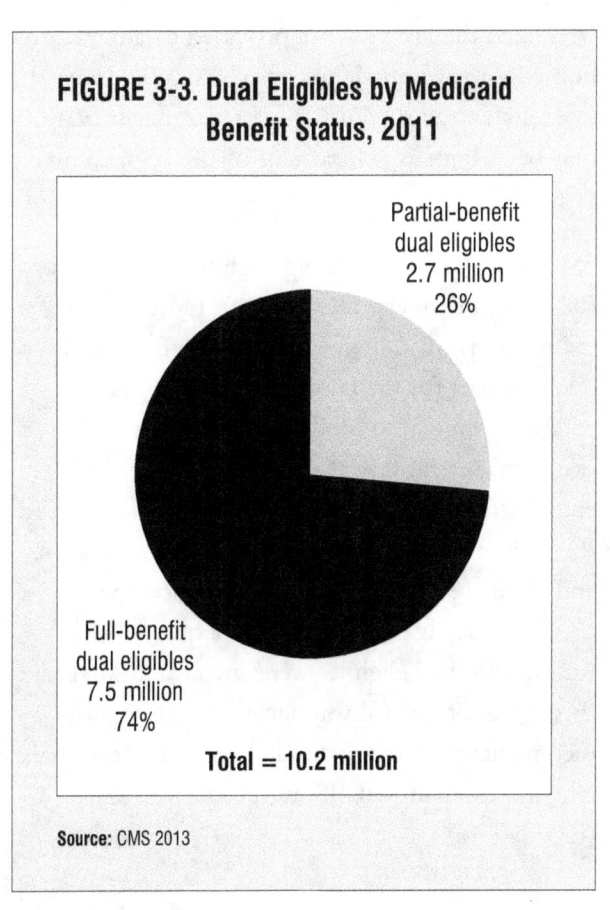

FIGURE 3-3. Dual Eligibles by Medicaid Benefit Status, 2011

Partial-benefit dual eligibles
2.7 million
26%

Full-benefit dual eligibles
7.5 million
74%

Total = 10.2 million

Source: CMS 2013

District of Columbia had this type of coverage (MACStats Table 11).

Medically needy eligibility. The medically needy option, offered by 32 states and the District of Columbia, enables states to cover persons with higher income who may have significant expenses for medical care or supportive services (MACStats Table 11). People with income above the medically needy threshold can deduct incurred expenses from their income—or spend down—below the financial eligibility threshold.[3] States may use different financial thresholds for medically needy eligibility and have the option to limit the Medicaid benefits package for these individuals.

Special income rule. States have the option to provide Medicaid benefits to people meeting special state income standards for nursing home residents, for participants in home and community-based waiver services (HCBS) programs—which serve people in the community who need the level of care provided by a nursing home—or for both. These special standards, used in 43 states and the District of Columbia in 2012, may be as high as 300 percent of the SSI benefit rate.

SSI is the primary Medicaid eligibility pathway for full-benefit dual eligibles. In 2007, more than half (56 percent) of individuals who were full-benefit dual eligibles for the entire year (all-year dual eligibles) came in to Medicaid through the SSI program. A relatively small percentage of dual eligibles (9 percent) were enrolled for full Medicaid through other poverty-related eligibility pathways, and about 12 percent came into Medicaid via a medically needy pathway. Nearly a quarter of full-benefit dual eligibles were enrolled in Medicaid through another pathway, including the special income limit for the institutionalized or individuals who are receiving HCBS waiver services (Figure 3-4).

Because the special income limit and medically needy pathways are used by people with high medical or LTSS needs, enrollees in these groups have much higher Medicaid spending, on average, than do dual eligibles who come in via the SSI or poverty-related pathways. All-year, full-benefit dually eligible individuals enrolled in Medicaid through a medically needy or special income pathway had average Medicaid costs of $36,085 and $28,680, respectively, in 2007, compared to average per capita spending of just about $8,000 for those enrolled through an SSI or poverty-related eligibility pathway (not shown).

Medicaid's Role for Dual Eligibles

Since Medicare is the primary payer for health care for dual eligibles, Medicaid acts as a secondary

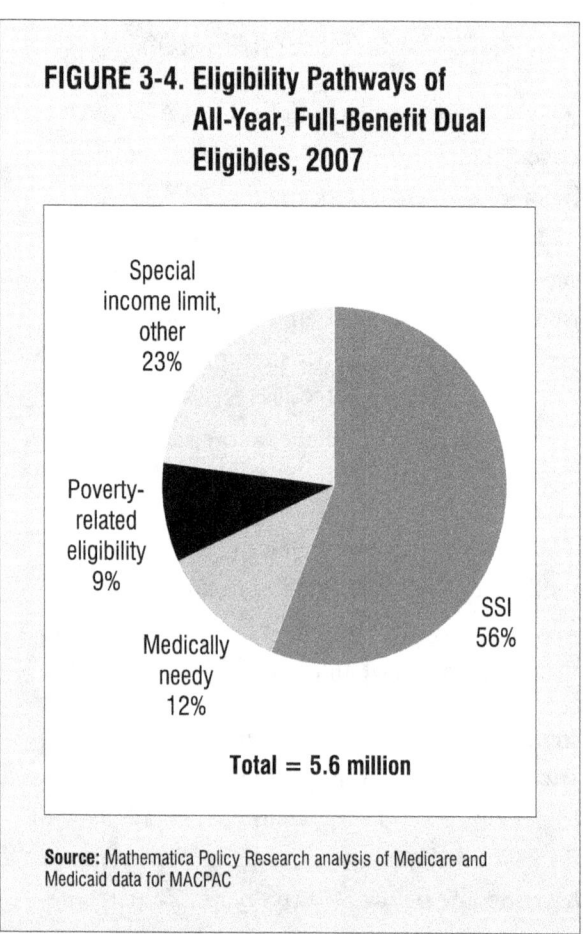

FIGURE 3-4. Eligibility Pathways of All-Year, Full-Benefit Dual Eligibles, 2007

- Special income limit, other 23%
- Poverty-related eligibility 9%
- Medically needy 12%
- SSI 56%

Total = 5.6 million

Source: Mathematica Policy Research analysis of Medicare and Medicaid data for MACPAC.

payer, filling in Medicare cost sharing and covering other acute care services not covered by Medicare. For example, Medicaid may cover acute care and post-acute services after the Medicare benefit is exhausted or if certain Medicare criteria are not met. Full-benefit dual eligibles are eligible for payment of any benefits covered under a state plan—if Medicare does not cover the service or if Medicare benefits have been exhausted—including certain mandatory federal benefits and any additional optional benefits that the state has decided to provide.[4]

Nationally, Medicaid spending on dual eligibles came to nearly $107 billion in 2007, including $75.1 billion on LTSS, $10.5 billion on Medicare premiums, and $21.4 billion on acute care services, including acute care services not covered by Medicare and Medicaid payments for Medicare cost sharing (which could not be disaggregated in the current analysis) (Figure 3-5).

Because Medicaid provides significant flexibility to states, Medicaid benefits for dual eligibles vary widely across the states. For example, some states impose much more restrictive clinical or functional eligibility requirements for nursing home services than others, limiting the number of people who are eligible to receive Medicaid-financed long-term nursing home care and the number eligible to receive services under HCBS waivers.

States have considerable flexibility under Medicaid to provide LTSS—both in institutional and in home and community-based settings—to adults age 65 and older who are frail or have disabilities and to non-elderly adults and children with disabilities who require supportive services. For people who have serious disabling conditions who meet state-based criteria for institutional care, Medicaid pays for supportive and skilled services in institutional settings, including nursing homes, ICFs/ID, and inpatient psychiatric facilities (for

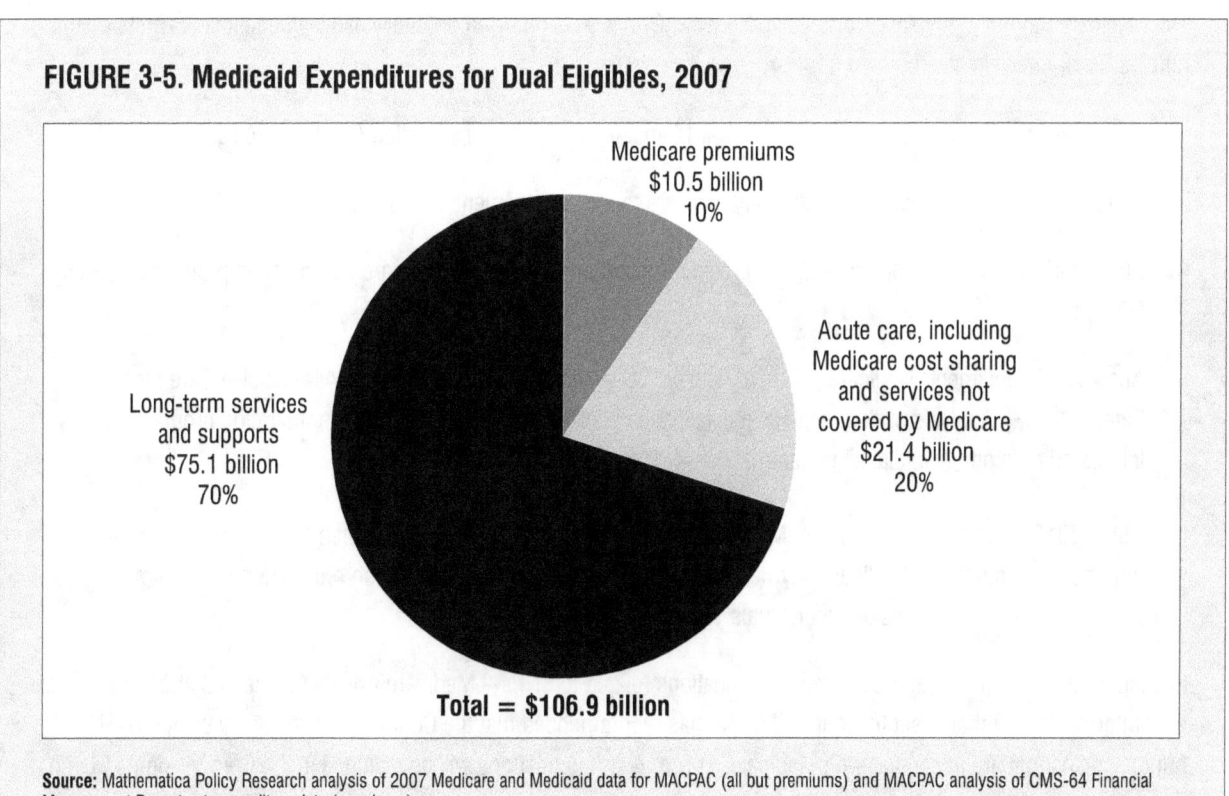

FIGURE 3-5. Medicaid Expenditures for Dual Eligibles, 2007

- Medicare premiums $10.5 billion 10%
- Acute care, including Medicare cost sharing and services not covered by Medicare $21.4 billion 20%
- Long-term services and supports $75.1 billion 70%

Total = $106.9 billion

Source: Mathematica Policy Research analysis of 2007 Medicare and Medicaid data for MACPAC (all but premiums) and MACPAC analysis of CMS-64 Financial Management Report net expenditure data (premiums)

people age 20 and younger and 65 and older). All states are required to provide home health benefits. Optional services include personal care attendant services, adult day health program services, and respite care. Care management is a covered service in Medicaid's home health benefit, in the personal care assistance benefits provided under a state plan, in HCBS waiver programs, and in the Program of All-inclusive Care for the Elderly (PACE). Many frail older adults and younger adults with disabilities receiving LTSS in Medicaid receive health and functional needs assessments, care plans, and care management services.

Medicaid benefits—those that are required to be provided (such as nursing facility services and home health) and those that are optional—must be provided on a statewide basis to everyone who is eligible for them. However, under waivers, states have substantial flexibility to target additional benefits and services to selected groups. The HCBS waiver program is the primary vehicle states use to finance non-institutional LTSS for people with disabilities. Under HCBS waivers, states can provide a wide range of services to enable persons with disabilities to achieve maximum independence in the community.

People receiving services under HCBS waivers often have unique constellations of needs that are very different from people with less severe disabilities living independently in the community. Individuals with a wide range of needs form this group, which includes people with intellectual disabilities, traumatic brain injury, physical disabilities, serious mental illness, and older adults who are frail or who have Alzheimer's disease or other cognitive limitations.

BOX 3-1. MedPAC's Recent Reports on People Who Are Dually Eligible for Medicare and Medicaid

The Medicare Payment Advisory Commission (MedPAC) has also reported on dually eligible beneficiaries in its recent reports. Their analysis has focused on:

- A profile of dual-eligible beneficiaries and their Medicare and Medicaid spending (MedPAC 2012a).

- Enrollment in integrated care programs and barriers to the development of integrated care (MedPAC 2010).

- Characteristics of managed care-based, provider-based, and fee-for-service care coordination programs (MedPAC 2011).

- Analysis of enrollment, Medicare payment, and quality measures in the Program of All-inclusive Care for the Elderly (PACE); analysis of dual-eligible special needs plans (D-SNPs); and CMS demonstration programs on integrated care and financial alignment. (MedPAC 2012b).

In its June 2012 Report to the Congress, MedPAC made recommendations related to the PACE program, including recommendations related to Medicare payments for PACE organizations. MedPAC also recommended changing the eligibility criteria for PACE to include individuals younger than 55.

In January 2013, MedPAC approved recommendations related to SNPs—Medicare Advantage plans that operate under a statutory authority that is set to expire. MedPAC has recommended that the Congress permanently extend D-SNPs, but only plans that are integrated with Medicaid. These recommendations will be included in the Commission's March 2013 Report to the Congress.

Depending on the needs and circumstances (e.g., availability of family members to provide assistance) of these individuals, the services provided under waivers vary widely and can include assistance with personal needs such as bathing, eating, and toileting, but may also include a broad range of supportive services that are related to maintaining function and maximum integration into the community. These may include supports for employment, adult day programs, transportation services, and habilitative services that allow a person with a disability to acquire or maintain life skills. States can also pay for housing to enable community living for people who would otherwise require an institutional level of care.

Waivers hold tremendous appeal for states because waivers enable them to annually budget for the number of persons who will be enrolled in the program and to establish participant waiting lists when that number is reached. As a result, some people who qualify for services may not receive them (Justice 2010). Services may be limited to specific groups (by type of disability, geographic region, or income, for example). Without federal minimum standards, some states have developed relatively comprehensive long-term care systems, while others offer relatively limited and fragmented care (Leutz 1999). As a result, low-income Medicare beneficiaries with disabilities may receive widely varying Medicaid assistance from state to state, and even within states if waiver services are not available statewide to all populations.

Dual Eligibles' Service Use and Spending across Both Programs

Dual eligibles vary widely in terms of their needs for medical care (whether they have serious acute or chronic conditions or multiple chronic conditions, for example) and their needs for LTSS. To illustrate the variation in care needs and the extent to which different dually eligible subpopulations rely on Medicare and Medicaid, this section examines the Medicare and Medicaid service use and spending of full-benefit dual eligibles, focusing on four subpopulations defined in terms of their use of Medicaid-financed LTSS. A recent analysis by Randall Brown and David Mann used similar categories (Brown and Mann 2012).

Dual-eligible subgroups

For this analysis, we took the full-benefit dual-eligible population that was enrolled in both Medicare and Medicaid for the entire year and divided the group into four mutually exclusive subgroups based on their use of Medicaid LTSS: an institutional users group, a group of people using HCBS waiver services, a group of people using state-plan LTSS only, and a group of people who do not use any Medicaid LTSS. Box 3-2 provides additional information on the data and methods.

Institutional group. The first subgroup includes dual eligibles who used any institutional services in Medicaid. This includes people who received Medicaid-financed nursing home services or LTSS in other institutional settings such as ICFs/ID. These individuals may also have used Medicaid HCBS under a waiver or regular Medicaid state plan rules.

HCBS waiver group. The second group includes people who received any services under Medicaid HCBS waivers. These individuals may have received state plan HCBS, such as home health care or personal care, but this category excludes anyone who received any Medicaid-financed institutional services during the year.

HCBS non-waiver group. The third group includes people who used regular state-plan

BOX 3-2. Methodology for the Analysis of the Dually Eligible Population

This analysis of dual eligibles' Medicare and Medicaid service use and spending is based on linked beneficiary-level data for 2007 from several sources, including the Medicaid Analytic eXtract (MAX) person summary file, Medicare Beneficiary Annual Summary File, and person summary files for Medicare Part D and Medicare Advantage. Individuals were identified as dually eligible if they were ever enrolled in both programs during the year, using indicators contained in the MAX data. Since enrollment status may vary during the year, individuals were classified as receiving full or partial Medicaid benefits based on their most recent month of dual eligibility.

To facilitate comparisons of annual spending across subgroups within the full-benefit dually eligible population, the information presented in this section and below is limited to people who were enrolled in both programs for the entire year (all-year enrollees), including people who were enrolled on January 1, 2007, but who died during the year.

Most dual eligibles—6.9 million, or more than three-fourths—were enrolled in both Medicare and Medicaid throughout the year, reflecting the stability of Medicaid coverage for older adults and non-elderly persons with disabilities: once enrolled in Medicaid, they tend to stay enrolled. The all-year dual-eligible population includes 5.6 million full-benefit dual eligibles and 1.3 million partial-benefit dual eligibles. About 2.1 million (23 percent) were enrolled for only part of the year (Figure 3-6).

We disaggregated the all-year, full-benefit dual-eligible population by their use of Medicaid LTSS. We created four distinct (non-overlapping) groups defined as follows: (1) institutional group, (2) HCBS waiver group, (3) non-waiver HCBS group, and (4) non-LTSS user group: people who did not use any Medicaid LTSS.

We included in our enrollment and expenditure estimates dual eligibles enrolled in Medicare or Medicaid managed care plans. The annual amount of the Medicare and Medicaid payments to these plans (the per enrollee capitation) is included in the spending data reported below, but information on the service use and expenditures of these plan enrollees (encounter data) is not reported because it was not available (Medicare) or was of unknown quality and completeness (Medicaid). Readers should note that MAX data are known to undercount total U.S. Medicaid spending relative to CMS-64 data submitted by states to obtain federal matching funds, with variation by state and type of service. Medicaid spending amounts presented in this chapter have not been adjusted to address this issue, as may be done in other MACPAC analyses. In addition, most figures exclude Medicaid payments for Medicare premiums, which are effectively reflected in the Medicare spending shown in the chapter.

Although Medicaid benefits and eligibility for low-income people with Medicare and patterns of use and spending vary widely across states, this chapter provides a national picture. The Commission will examine state-level differences and their impacts in future reports.

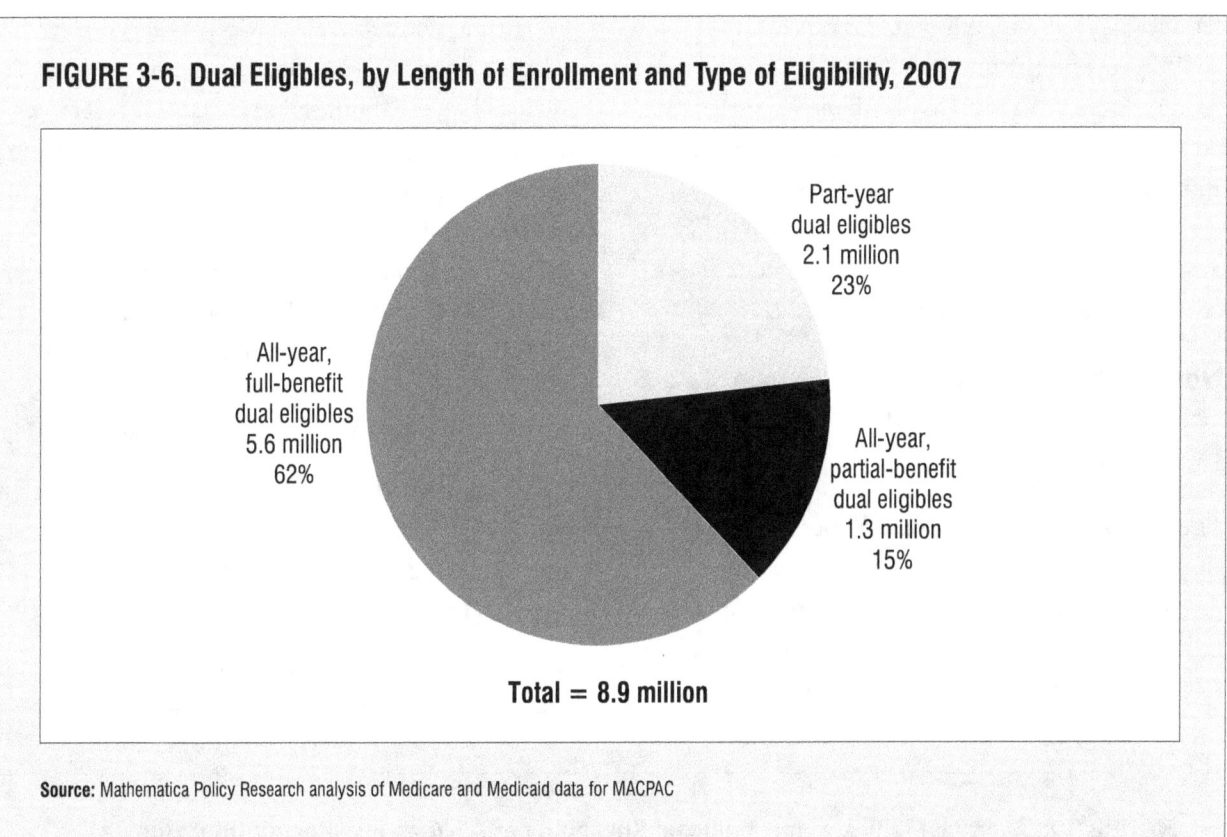

FIGURE 3-6. Dual Eligibles, by Length of Enrollment and Type of Eligibility, 2007

- Part-year dual eligibles: 2.1 million, 23%
- All-year, partial-benefit dual eligibles: 1.3 million, 15%
- All-year, full-benefit dual eligibles: 5.6 million, 62%

Total = 8.9 million

Source: Mathematica Policy Research analysis of Medicare and Medicaid data for MACPAC

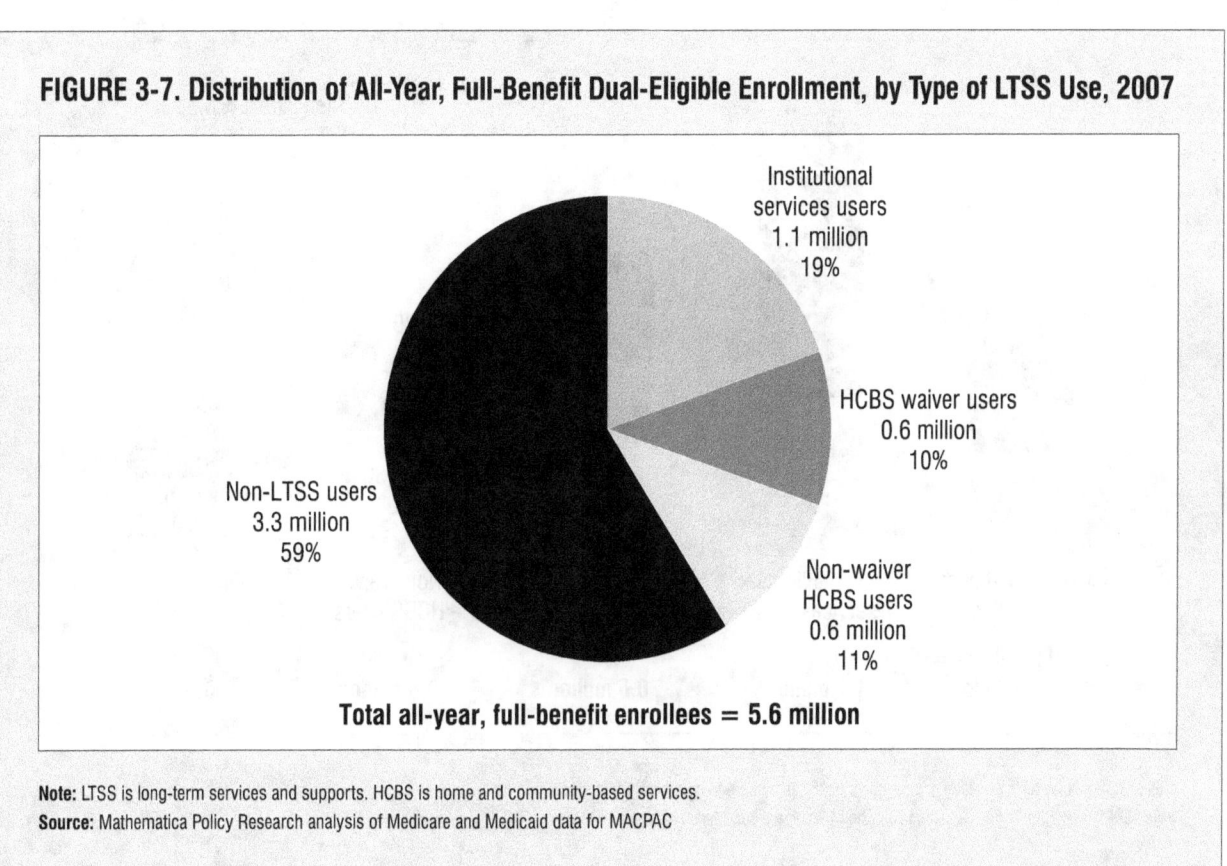

FIGURE 3-7. Distribution of All-Year, Full-Benefit Dual-Eligible Enrollment, by Type of LTSS Use, 2007

- Institutional services users: 1.1 million, 19%
- HCBS waiver users: 0.6 million, 10%
- Non-waiver HCBS users: 0.6 million, 11%
- Non-LTSS users: 3.3 million, 59%

Total all-year, full-benefit enrollees = 5.6 million

Note: LTSS is long-term services and supports. HCBS is home and community-based services.
Source: Mathematica Policy Research analysis of Medicare and Medicaid data for MACPAC

services in Medicaid, but who did not use any HCBS waiver or institutional LTSS. People in this group may have used state plan benefits such as home health care, personal care attendant services, and adult day health program services that are generally available to persons who are frail or have disabilities, but who do not necessarily meet the criteria for admission to a nursing home.

Non-LTSS user group. The fourth group includes dually eligible individuals who did not use any Medicaid LTSS.

The analysis shows that nearly 30 percent of all-year, full-benefit dual eligibles had serious disabilities and were eligible for nursing facility or other institutional care under Medicaid—including 19 percent who received institutional services and 10 percent who received services under Medicaid HCBS waivers. In addition, 11 percent used some Medicaid HCBS, but used only state-plan services that do not require an individual to meet a nursing home level of need. However, the majority of full-benefit dual eligibles (59 percent) did not use any Medicaid-financed LTSS (Figure 3-7). If partial-benefit dual eligibles who were enrolled in both programs for the entire year are included in the analysis, about two-thirds of dual eligibles (67 percent) did not use Medicaid-funded LTSS (not shown).

Variation in spending across dual-eligible subgroups

Average total program expenditures rise steadily with LTSS needs and types of service use

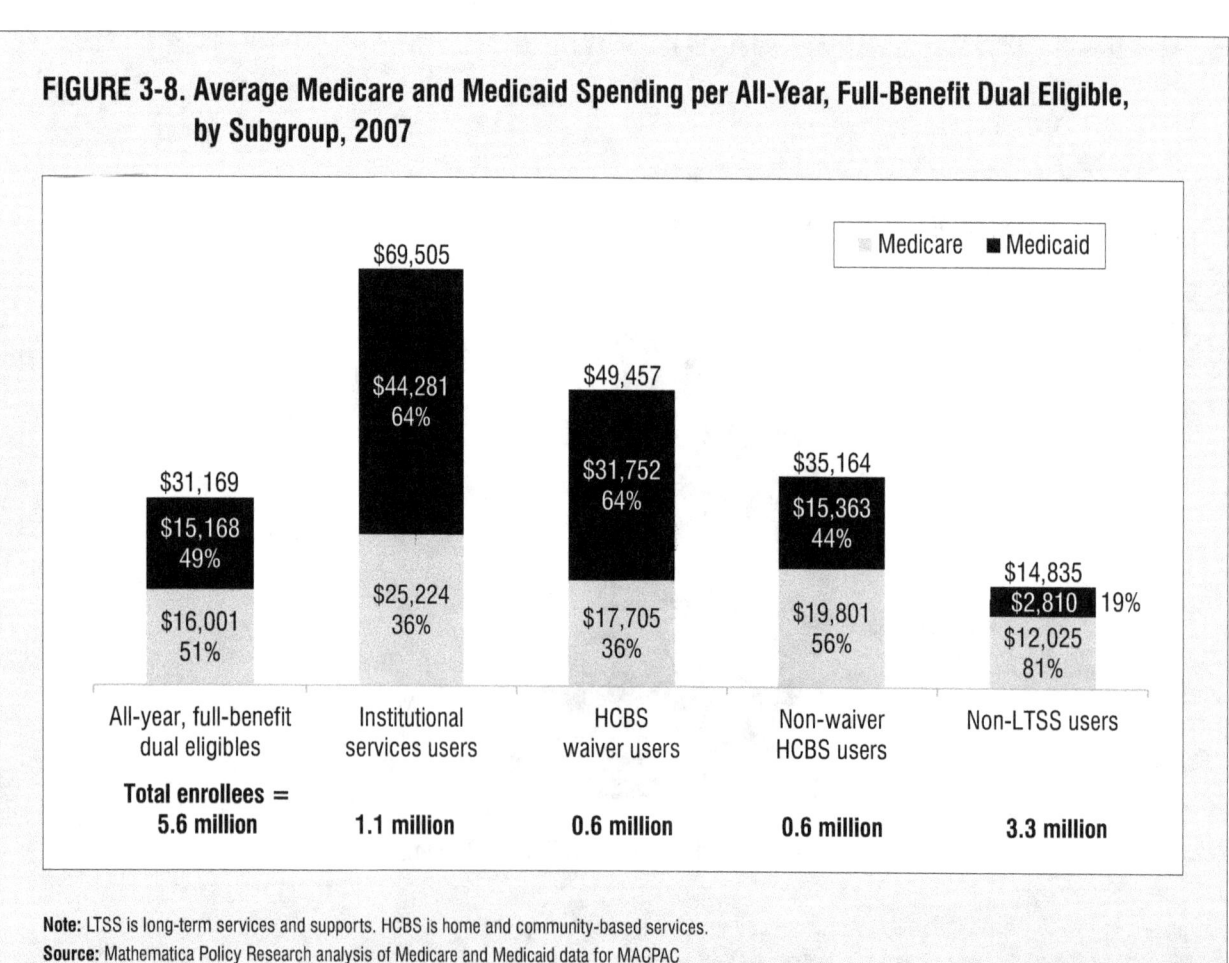

FIGURE 3-8. Average Medicare and Medicaid Spending per All-Year, Full-Benefit Dual Eligible, by Subgroup, 2007

Note: LTSS is long-term services and supports. HCBS is home and community-based services.
Source: Mathematica Policy Research analysis of Medicare and Medicaid data for MACPAC

CHAPTER 3: THE ROLES OF MEDICARE AND MEDICAID FOR A DIVERSE DUAL-ELIGIBLE POPULATION | MACPAC

TABLE 3-1. Medicare and Medicaid Spending per All-Year, Full-Benefit Dual Eligible, by Type of Service, 2007

Distribution of spending per enrollee by program and service category	Institutional services users		All-Year, Full-Benefit Dual Eligibles					
			HCBS waiver users		Non-waiver HCBS users		Non-LTSS users	
Medicare inpatient	$7,721	11.1%	$4,404	8.9%	$5,755	16.4%	$2,806	18.9%
Medicaid inpatient	588	0.8	278	0.6	500	1.4	203	1.4
Medicare outpatient, physician, & other acute	6,628	9.5	5,020	10.2	6,276	17.8	3,627	24.5
Medicaid outpatient, physician, & other acute	1,736	2.5	2,304	4.7	2,552	7.3	1,319	8.9
Medicare drugs	4,791	6.9	4,831	9.8	4,831	13.7	3,253	21.9
Medicaid drugs	122	0.2	152	0.3	188	0.5	107	0.7
Medicare skilled nursing facility	4,292	6.2	493	1.0	285	0.8	162	1.1
Medicaid nursing facility or other institution	40,284	58.0	0	0.0	0	0.0	0	0.0
Medicare home health	381	0.5	1,664	3.4	1,405	4.0	507	3.4
Medicaid home health	187	0.3	536	1.1	1,834	5.2	0	0.0
Medicaid HCBS, other than home health	1,117	1.6	27,978	56.6	9,653	27.5	0	0.0
Medicare capitated payments	1,411	2.0	1,293	2.6	1,249	3.6	1,670	11.3
Medicaid capitated payments	247	0.4	504	1.0	636	1.8	1,181	8.0
Combined program spending per enrollee	$69,505	100%	$49,457	100%	$35,164	100%	$14,835	100%
Medicaid spending per enrollee	$44,281	64%	$31,752	64%	$15,363	44%	$2,810	19%
Medicare spending per enrollee	$25,224	36%	$17,705	36%	$19,801	56%	$12,025	81%
Total program spending (billions)	$74.4		$28.5		$22.0		$49.0	
Number of enrollees (millions)	1.2		0.5		0.5		3.3	

Source: Mathematica Policy Research analysis of Medicare and Medicaid data for MACPAC

(Table 3-1, Figure 3-8). For each of the three LTSS user subgroups, the large majority of Medicaid spending was for long-term care services—with these expenditures far surpassing spending on any other Medicare- or Medicaid-financed service (Table 3-1, Figure 3-9).

Spending among non-LTSS users. The largest subgroup, comprised of dually eligible individuals who did not use LTSS, had the lowest total spending, with combined per capita Medicare and Medicaid spending of $14,835—the large majority of it (81 percent) in Medicare (Figure 3-8). This subgroup had the lowest use of Medicare-covered services and the lowest per capita spending in Medicare. For example, only 19 percent used any inpatient hospital services during the year (compared to 41 percent of the institutional subgroup), 77 percent used Medicare physician services, 63 percent used outpatient hospital services, and 91 percent used prescription drugs (Figure 3-10).

People in the non-LTSS user subgroup also had by far the lowest spending in Medicaid. Only a small percentage used any wraparound services in Medicaid (only 12 percent used any dental services under Medicaid, 10 percent used transportation services, and 11 percent used Medicaid psychiatric services). Most of the Medicaid spending for these non-LTSS users was for services covered by Medicare (e.g., inpatient hospital, outpatient hospital, and physician services) (Table 3-1).

Spending among non-waiver HCBS users. Dual eligibles who used state-plan LTSS only (the non-waiver HCBS subgroup) had average combined program spending ($35,164 per capita)

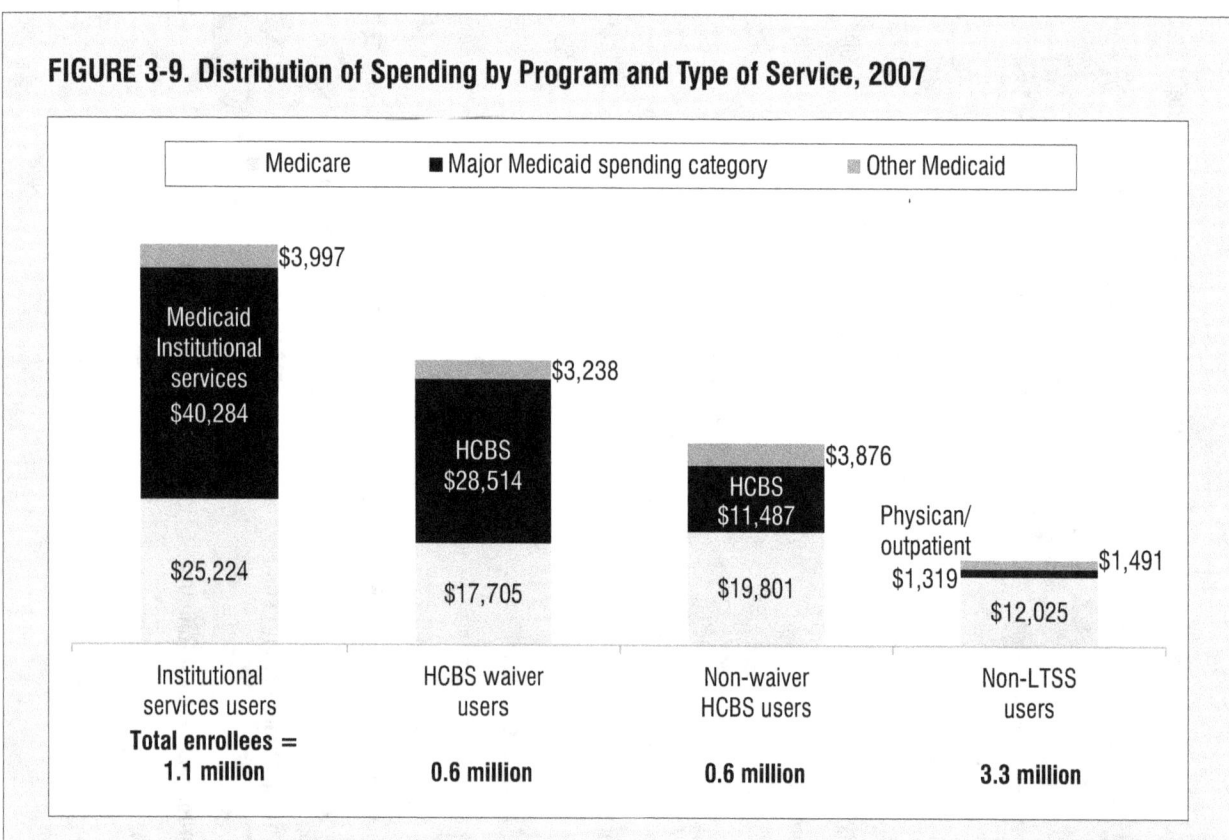

FIGURE 3-9. Distribution of Spending by Program and Type of Service, 2007

Notes: LTSS is long-term services and supports. HCBS is home and community-based services. The major Medicaid spending category is the largest category of spending by type of service. See Table 3-1 for additional detail on spending by type of service.

Source: Mathematica Policy Research analysis of Medicare and Medicaid data for MACPAC

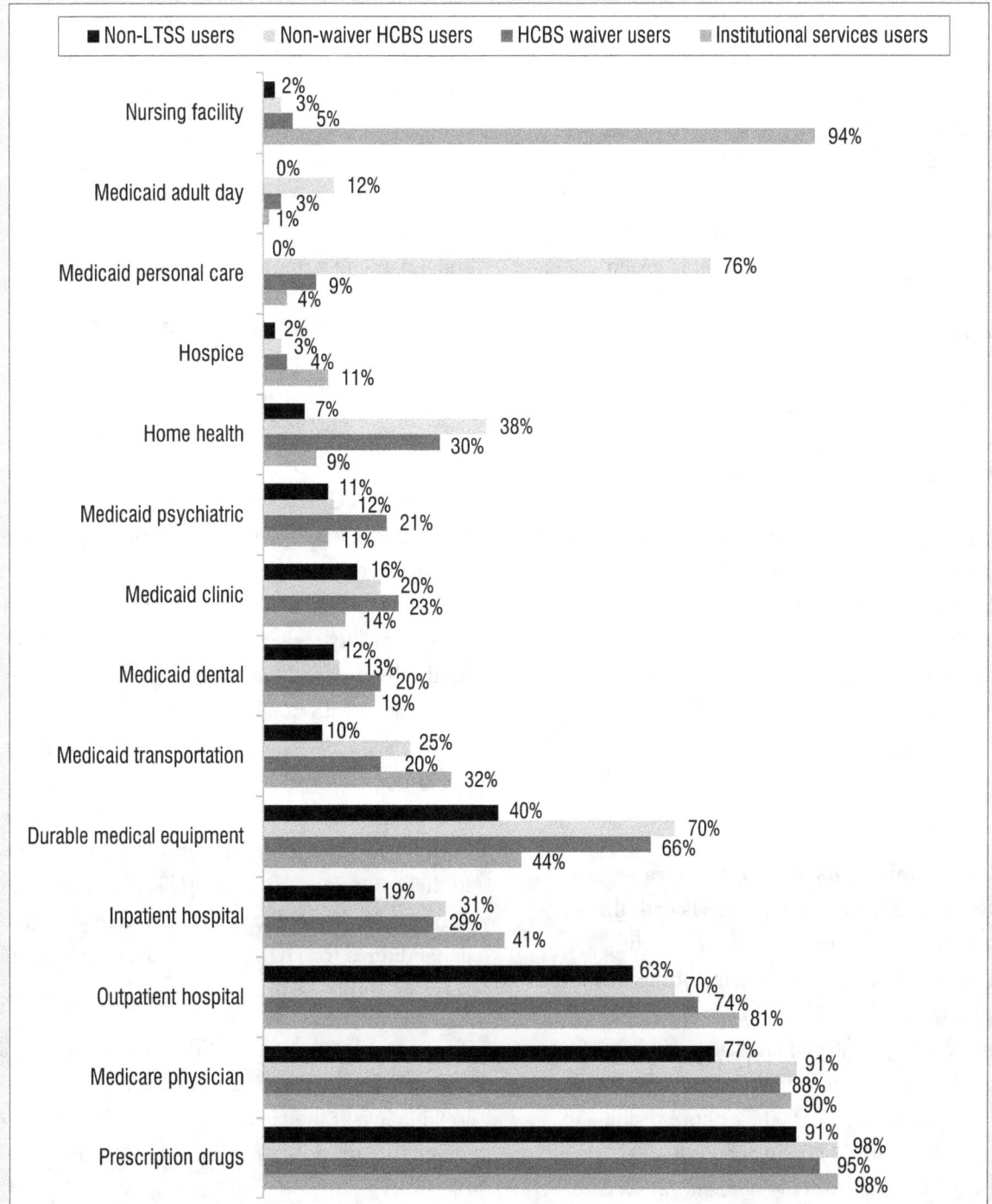

FIGURE 3-10. Percentage of All-Year, Full-Benefit Dual Eligibles Using Selected Services, by Subgroup, 2007

more than twice as high as the non-LTSS user group, with spending roughly evenly split between Medicare and Medicaid (Figure 3-8). Most of the difference in spending between these groups was accounted for by much higher Medicaid spending in the non-waiver HCBS group compared to the non-LTSS user group ($15,363 vs. $2,810), but their Medicare spending was also higher. Most of the Medicaid spending ($11,487 of the $15,363) for these dual eligibles was for LTSS (Figure 3-9), including spending on state-plan personal care (used by 76 percent of people in this group), Medicaid home health services (used by 23 percent, not shown), and state-plan adult day services (used by 12 percent). They also had somewhat higher use of some Medicaid wraparound services, including non-emergency transportation (used by a quarter of dual eligibles in this subgroup).

Dually eligible individuals in the non-waiver HCBS subgroup had higher average spending in Medicare ($19,801) than dual eligibles in the non-LTSS user group ($12,025). Correspondingly, they had higher use rates for Medicare services, including inpatient hospitalization (31 vs. 19 percent for the non-LTSS users), physician services (91 vs. 77 percent), and prescription drugs (98 vs. 91 percent), and higher spending on these services (Table 3-1).

Spending among users of HCBS waiver services. Dually eligible individuals with the most significant disabilities—who met the criteria for admission to a nursing home, ICF/ID, or psychiatric facility—had still higher average combined program spending (nearly $50,000 for dual eligibles receiving services under HCBS waivers, and nearly $70,000 for those residing in institutions), with Medicaid accounting for the majority of these costs (64 percent, on average) (Figure 3-8)

Dual eligibles using HCBS waiver services had Medicare spending that was slightly lower than Medicare spending for the non-waiver HCBS group. Nearly all of the Medicaid spending for people in the HCBS waiver subgroup, and 56 percent of their combined Medicare and Medicaid spending, was for the waiver services themselves, although there was some very modest spending for state-plan LTSS, mainly home health (Figure 3-9, Table 3-1). These dual eligibles also had higher rates of use of Medicaid-financed services, including psychiatric services (21 percent) and clinic services (23 percent), compared to the state-plan LTSS user group.

Spending among users of institutional services. The subgroup of dual eligibles using institutional LTSS had the highest average spending in Medicare and, correspondingly, the highest rates of medical care service use. Among dual eligibles who received LTSS in institutional settings, 41 percent used inpatient hospital services and 81 percent used hospital outpatient services. Ninety-four percent used nursing facility services (the remaining 6 percent used other institutional services, mostly facilities for persons with intellectual disabilities). Spending on Medicaid institutional services accounted for the large majority (90 percent) of all Medicaid spending and most (58 percent) of total program spending on this group (Figure 3-9). Since some in the institutional user group likely resided in the community during the year, there were also modest expenditures for HCBS, both waiver and state plan services (Table 3-1).

There are also significant differences in service use and spending within these groups. For example, looking just at the HCBS waiver services group—which is comprised of roughly equal numbers of adults younger than 65 and those age 65 and older—the mix of services used varies significantly across older and younger program participants. Utilization rates for HCBS waiver residential care, targeted case management, dental care, and psychiatric services in Medicaid are significantly higher for non-elderly than for HCBS waiver participants who are age 65 and older, suggesting that non-elderly dual eligibles receiving services under HCBS waivers, on average, have far different needs than dual-eligible waiver participants age 65 and older (Figure 3-11).

Similarly, for people using institutional services in Medicaid, there are wide differences in spending by age, suggesting that those under age 65 have different kinds of care needs. Medicaid spending was substantially higher for non-elderly dual eligibles who use institutional LTSS than for their counterparts age 65 and older, for example (Figure 3-12). Most dual eligibles who receive institutional services received services in nursing homes (99 percent of persons age 65 and older and 67 percent of the non-elderly), but 30 percent of the non-elderly received services in ICFs/ID (not shown).

The fact that these groups have very different levels and kinds of needs, as reflected in patterns of service use and spending, suggests that different approaches may be needed to improve the way the programs work for distinct dual-eligible subpopulations. To be successful, providers and plans will need knowledge and understanding of particular populations, including unique expertise serving people with serious disabilities who receive LTSS under HCBS waiver programs designed to promote independence and community integration.

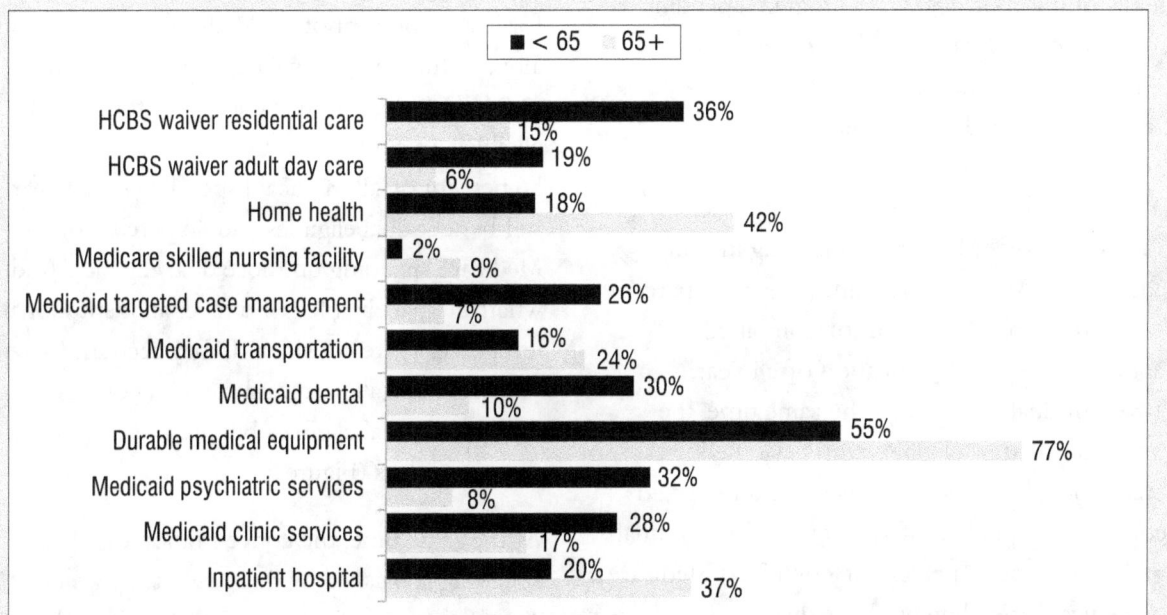

FIGURE 3-11. Percentage of All-Year, Full-Benefit Dual Eligible HCBS Waiver Participants Using Selected Medicare- and Medicaid-Financed Services, by Age, 2007

Note: Data are for all-year, full-benefit dually eligible individuals in HCBS waiver user subgroup. Unless otherwise indicated, Medicaid services are state plan services. Not all service use is reported. Total use of a service like home health or durable medical equipment can be higher because (1) services may be funded under waivers (not shown here) as well as under a state plan and (2) services provided under capitated managed care arrangements are excluded.
Source: Mathematica Policy Research analysis of Medicare and Medicaid data for MACPAC

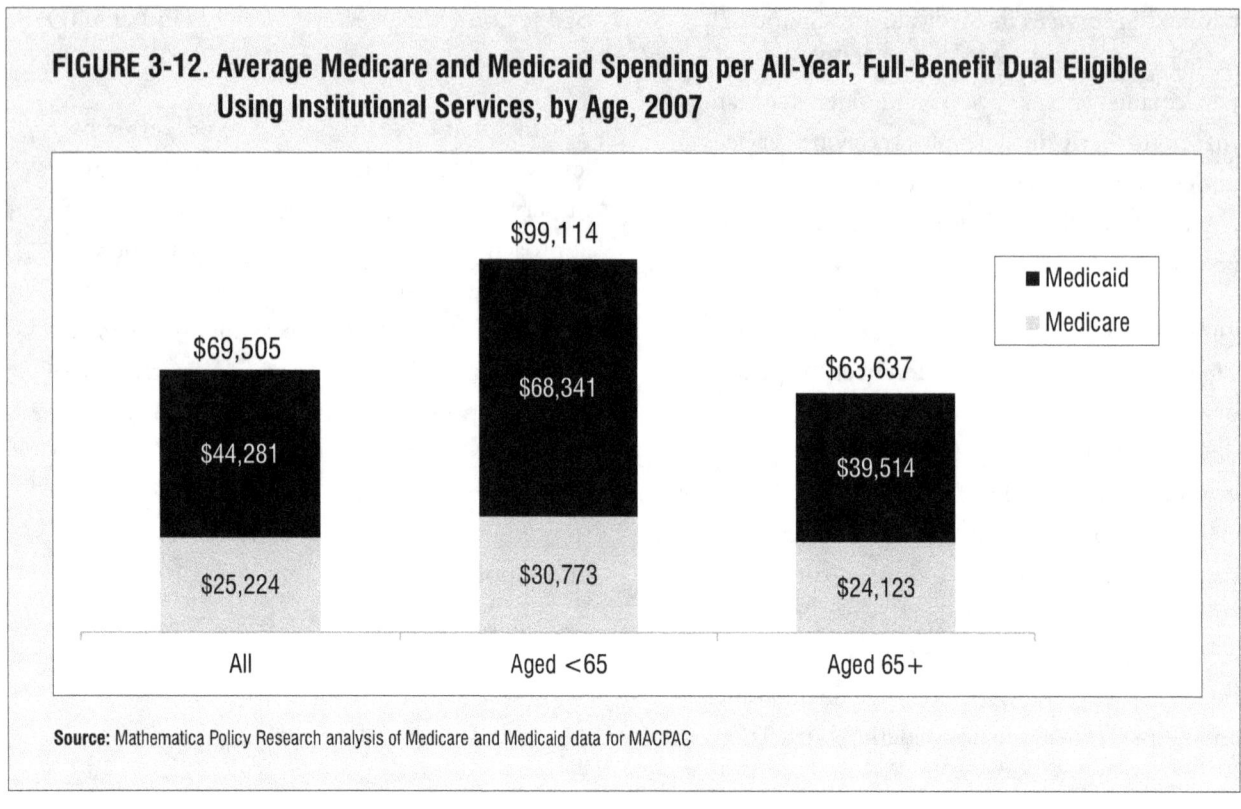

FIGURE 3-12. Average Medicare and Medicaid Spending per All-Year, Full-Benefit Dual Eligible Using Institutional Services, by Age, 2007

Source: Mathematica Policy Research analysis of Medicare and Medicaid data for MACPAC

Aggregate program spending by subgroup

The distribution of aggregate program spending—for combined program spending on dual eligibles and for Medicare and Medicaid separately—illustrates the overall consequences of these different patterns of use for public spending on dual eligibles. For example, institutional users, who have the highest average spending in both Medicare and Medicaid, account for just 19 percent of enrollment but 43 percent of combined spending on the total population of all-year, full-benefit dual eligibles. At the same time, the large group of dual eligibles who have the lowest average spending in both Medicare and Medicaid account for 59 percent of all-year, full-benefit dual eligibles, but just 28 percent of combined Medicare and Medicaid spending on those dual eligibles (Figure 3-13).

Considering each program's expenditures on dually eligible individuals highlights the differences among subgroups. For example, non-LTSS users who account for 59 percent of enrollees have relatively low spending in Medicaid and account for just 11 percent of all Medicaid spending on all-year, full-benefit dual eligibles but a third of Medicare program spending on those dual eligibles. In contrast, institutional users account for 56 percent of all Medicaid spending on all-year, full-benefit dual eligibles and 44 percent of Medicare spending on those dual eligibles. And, when all dual eligibles who meet an institutional level of care are considered, they account for 78 percent of all Medicaid spending on all-year, full-benefit dual eligibles but are just 29 percent of those enrollees (Figure 3-13).

At the same time, the concentration of Medicaid spending is masked by these subgroup averages. The 10 percent of all-year, full-benefit dually eligible individuals with the highest spending in Medicaid accounts for 51 percent of all Medicaid spending on those dual eligibles but just 13 percent of all Medicare spending on those dual eligibles

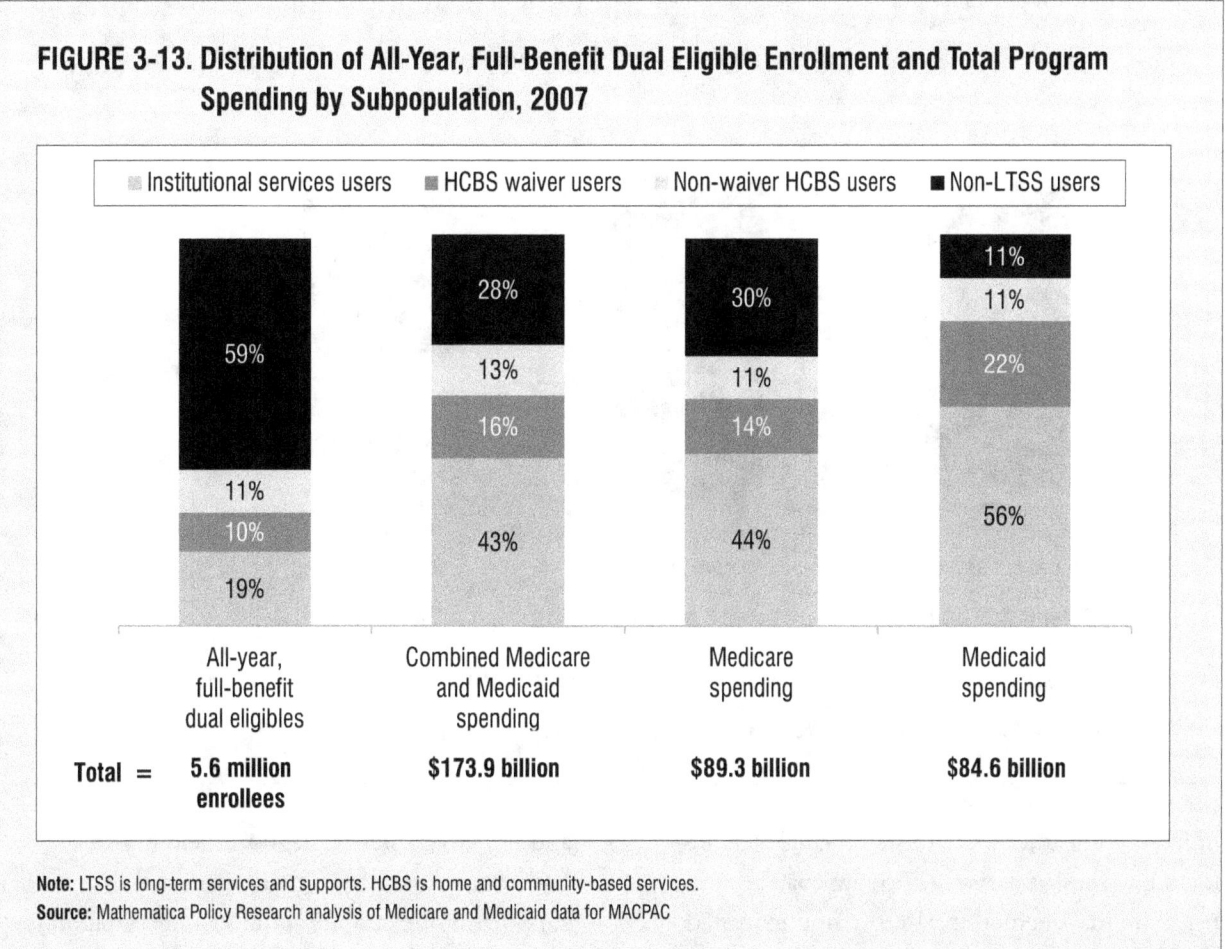

FIGURE 3-13. Distribution of All-Year, Full-Benefit Dual Eligible Enrollment and Total Program Spending by Subpopulation, 2007

Note: LTSS is long-term services and supports. HCBS is home and community-based services.
Source: Mathematica Policy Research analysis of Medicare and Medicaid data for MACPAC

(Figure 3-14). The highest cost dual eligibles in Medicaid had average total spending of about $100,000 in 2007—the large majority of it in Medicaid. Additional analysis is needed to better understand the LTSS needs of these beneficiaries and whether more appropriate and cost-effective approaches to service delivery can be developed for them.

Looking Forward

This use and spending profile begins to provide a picture of the diversity of the dual-eligible population. The wide variation in service use and spending implies that different approaches will be needed to address the distinct challenges faced by unique subgroups. For some groups, spending is mostly for LTSS designed to achieve independence and community living. Efforts to improve their care will need to focus on the management and coordination of unique constellations of LTSS, many of which are nonmedical. For others, service delivery improvement should more likely focus on the management of medical and behavioral health services and linkages to social services. For the large group of dual eligibles who have modest spending in Medicaid, the focus may need to be on Medicare strategies, access to wraparound benefits in Medicaid, and the impact of Medicaid policies for paying Medicare cost sharing on access to care.

In future work, the Commission will examine options for improving care and services for dual eligibles and the implications for both Medicare and Medicaid. The Commission will assess the evidence on a variety of interventions designed to

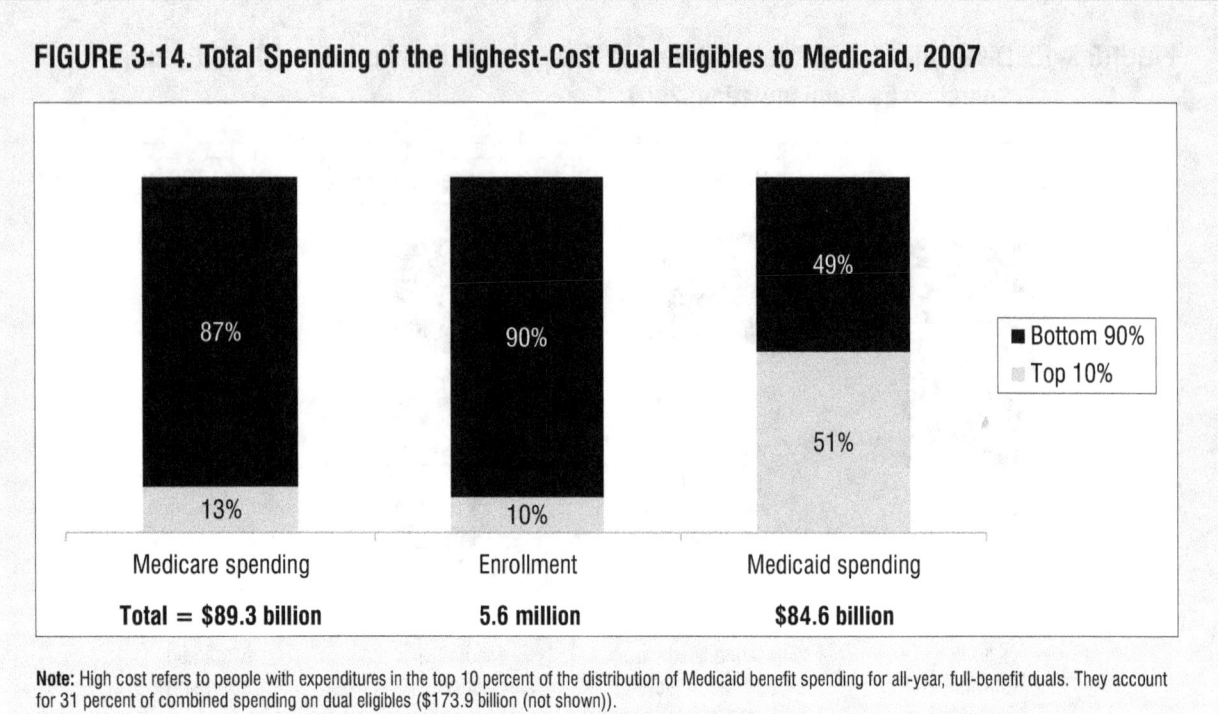

FIGURE 3-14. Total Spending of the Highest-Cost Dual Eligibles to Medicaid, 2007

Note: High cost refers to people with expenditures in the top 10 percent of the distribution of Medicaid benefit spending for all-year, full-benefit duals. They account for 31 percent of combined spending on dual eligibles ($173.9 billion (not shown)).
Source: Mathematica Policy Research analysis of Medicare and Medicaid data for MACPAC

improve care and reduce costs for dual eligibles, including fee-for-service (FFS) approaches (e.g. care management programs) and managed care approaches (e.g., provider-based programs such as PACE— which enrolls older adults with significant disabilities—and insurance-based models such as fully integrated special needs plans for dual eligibles). The Commission will follow with interest the design, implementation, and operation of new integrated care models under the Centers for Medicare & Medicaid Services financial alignment demonstrations. Moving forward, the Commission plans to:

Continue to assess the diverse needs and circumstances of dual eligibles and opportunities to improve care and services. In future work, the Commission will explore opportunities for program improvement for different segments of the dually eligible population. Evaluating approaches to reform will depend on a richer description of dual-eligible subpopulations, including information on health and functional status, diagnoses and health conditions, and living situation and family supports. For example, additional information is needed to understand the characteristics of the non-LTSS users and whether they have multiple or severe chronic illnesses or other characteristics associated with their service needs, including needs for care management.

Since the fastest growing segment of the dually eligible population is the non-elderly population, more attention may be needed to understand Medicaid's role for these dual eligibles. This segment includes people with intellectual disabilities, serious mental illness, and a wide range of physical disabilities and chronic conditions requiring ongoing care and supportive services. The analysis of service use and spending provided here leaves out a number of factors that would help deepen the understanding of the need for and design of policy reforms, including information on the number and severity of chronic and acute conditions (mental health needs, for example).

The Commission also plans to explore the service utilization of the large group of dual eligibles who do not use LTSS (who are relatively low cost to Medicaid) to better understand what Medicaid services they are accessing and what their unmet needs may be. The Commission will also examine the service needs, use, and spending of non-elderly dual eligibles who are under age 65 and have intellectual disabilities, and dual eligibles with severe mental illness.

Examine the factors that contribute to high spending and assess opportunities for savings. The Commission is interested in understanding the factors that contribute to high spending and whether there are opportunities to reduce spending without harming the quality of care or quality of life for dually eligible enrollees. The Commission will examine approaches such as those designed to reduce potentially avoidable hospitalizations of nursing home residents, integrated financing and delivery approaches in managed care, and FFS care management approaches.

Examine state variation and the impact of state policy choices. The Commission will also assess the extent to which access to Medicare-covered services for dual eligibles is affected by Medicaid policy choices. The analysis presented in this chapter focuses on national estimates of dual eligibles' service use and spending, to highlight distinct subgroups. But Medicaid programs vary widely in terms of covered benefits (for example, the scope of state plan HCBS provided) and payment policies (such as the adequacy of nursing home payment rates). These state policy choices may affect access to care and quality of care for dual eligibles, and potentially also affect dual eligibles' use and spending in Medicare.

As a first step in understanding the extent of state variation and its impact, the Commission will undertake an assessment of Medicaid policies for paying Medicare cost sharing and their impact on access to care. Although a number of factors may limit access to Medicare-covered services for low-income Medicare beneficiaries (residence in medically underserved areas, for example), a 2003 report to the Congress from the U.S. Department of Health and Human Services documented that access to care for dually eligible individuals was lower where Medicaid payments for Medicare cost sharing were lower, with especially large gaps in access to mental health providers in states that did not pay Medicare cost sharing in full (Thompson 2003). The Commission is interested in an updated assessment of the impact of these Medicaid payment policies.

Conclusion

The 10.2 million people who are dually eligible for Medicare and Medicaid receive a good deal of policy attention because they account for a relatively small share of enrollees in each program but account for a disproportionately large share of the expenditures in each program. Because of substantial or complex needs, dual eligibles often require a broad range of services and therefore rely on both programs. But the mix and intensity of services used—and the role each program plays—varies across subpopulations, suggesting that an array of approaches will be needed to address the distinct challenges of unique subgroups within the diverse dual-eligible populations. Understanding the service use and spending of key subpopulations is essential to identifying policy priorities and evaluating policy proposals. The Commission will explore policy options to address the diverse needs of the nation's dual-eligible populations in future work.

Endnotes

1 Dual eligibles who are under age 65 and are enrolled in Medicare as a result of a serious disability are typically enrolled in the Social Security Disability Insurance program or are adult children with disabilities or widows who qualify through other disability-related pathways to Social Security and Medicare.

2 The 209(b) option allows states to use their 1972 state assistance eligibility rules in determining eligibility for persons age 65 and older instead of federal SSI rules. However, a state using its 1972 income or resource thresholds must also allow people to deduct health care expenses from income in determining eligibility.

3 Historically, an individual with income even $1 above the threshold in a state without a medically needy program would be ineligible for coverage. However, Qualified Income Trusts were established to permit people with income above the financial eligibility threshold to put those resources in a trust to be used to offset future Medicaid expenses, thus establishing financial eligibility for Medicaid.

4 Under Medicaid, all states cover a minimum set of benefits including physician services, inpatient and outpatient hospital care, laboratory and x-ray services, home health care, and nursing home care. States have the option of covering additional services—such as prescription drugs and HCBS (including case management) for adults age 65 and older who are frail and persons with disabilities—and have broad discretion to determine the scope of those benefits.

References

Brown, R., and D.R. Mann. 2012. *Best bets for reducing Medicare costs for dual eligible beneficiaries: Assessing the evidence.* Washington, DC: Kaiser Family Foundation. http://www.kff.org/medicare/upload/8353.pdf.

Centers for Medicare & Medicaid Services (CMS), U.S. Department of Health and Human Services. 2011. *Medicare-Medicaid Coordination Office FY 2011 report to the Congress.* Baltimore, MD: CMS. http://www.cms.gov/Medicare-Medicaid-Coordination/Medicare-and-Medicaid-Coordination/Medicare-Medicaid-Coordination-Office/Downloads/MMCO_2011_RTC.pdf.

Centers for Medicare & Medicaid Services (CMS), U.S. Department of Health and Human Services. 2013. *Data Analysis Brief: Medicare-Medicaid dual enrollment from 2006 through 2011.* Baltimore, MD: CMS. http://www.cms.gov/Medicare-Medicaid-Coordination/Medicare-and-Medicaid-Coordination/Medicare-Medicaid-Coordination-Office/Downloads/Dual_Enrollment_2006-2011_Final_Document.pdf.

Coughlin, T.A., T. Waidmann, L. Phadera, et al. 2012. *The diversity of dual eligible beneficiaries: An examination of services and spending for people eligible for both Medicaid and Medicare.* Washington, DC: Kaiser Commission on Medicaid and the Uninsured. http://www.kff.org/medicaid/7895.cfm.

Justice, D. 2010. *Implementing the Affordable Care Act: New options for Medicaid home and community based services.* Washington, DC: National Academy of State Health Policy. http://www.nashp.org/sites/default/files/LTSS_SCAN-FINAL-9-29-10.PDF.

Leutz, W. 1999. Policy choices for Medicaid and Medicare waivers. *Gerontologist* 39, no. 1: 86–93.

Master, R.J. 2012. Realizing the promise of integrated care for the dual eligibles. *Health Affairs blog*, October 22, 2012.

Master, R.J, and C. Eng. 2001. Integrating acute and long-term care for high-cost populations. *Health Affairs* 20, no. 6: 161–172.

Medicare Payment Advisory Commission, (MedPAC). 2012a. *A databook: health care spending and the Medicare program.* Washington, DC: MedPAC.

Medicare Payment Advisory Commission, (MedPAC). 2012b. *Report to the Congress: Medicare and the health care delivery system.* Washington, DC: MedPAC.

Medicare Payment Advisory Commission, (MedPAC). 2011. *Report to the Congress: Medicare and the health care delivery system.* Washington, DC: MedPAC.

Medicare Payment Advisory Commission, (MedPAC). 2010. *Report to the Congress: Aligning incentives in Medicare.* Washington, DC: MedPAC.

Thompson, T. 2003. *Report to the Congress on state payment limitations for Medicare cost sharing.* Washington, DC: U.S. Department of Health and Human Services.

Whitelaw, N., and G. Warden. 1999. Reexamining the delivery system as part of Medicare reform. *Health Affairs* 18, no. 1: 132–143.

MACStats: Medicaid and CHIP Program Statistics

MACPAC | REPORT TO THE CONGRESS ON MEDICAID AND CHIP

MACStats Table of Contents

Overview 74

TABLE 1.	Medicaid and CHIP Enrollment as a Percentage of the U.S. Population, 2012 75
TABLE 2.	Medicaid Enrollment by State and Selected Characteristics, FY 2010 (thousands) 76
TABLE 3.	CHIP Enrollment by State, FY 2012 78
TABLE 4.	Child Enrollment in Medicaid-Financed Coverage by State, and CHIP-Financed Coverage by State and Family Income, FY 2011 80
TABLE 5.	Child Enrollment in Separate CHIP Programs by State and Managed Care Participation, FY 2012 82
TABLE 6.	Medicaid Spending by State, Category, and Source of Funds, FY 2012 (millions) 84
TABLE 7.	Total Medicaid Benefit Spending by State and Category, FY 2012 (millions) 86
TABLE 8.	CHIP Spending by State, FY 2012 (millions) 88
TABLE 9.	Medicaid and CHIP Income Eligibility Levels as a Percentage of the Federal Poverty Level for Children and Pregnant Women by State, February 2013 90
TABLE 10.	Medicaid Income Eligibility Levels as a Percentage of the Federal Poverty Level for Non-Aged, Non-Disabled, Non-Pregnant Adults by State, January 2013 94
TABLE 11.	Medicaid Income Eligibility Levels as a Percentage of the Federal Poverty Level for Individuals Age 65 and Older and Persons with Disabilities by State, 2012 98
TABLE 12.	Mandatory and Optional Medicaid Benefits 100
TABLE 13.	Maximum Allowable Medicaid Premiums and Cost Sharing, FY 2013 103
TABLE 14.	Federal Medical Assistance Percentages (FMAPs) and Enhanced FMAPs (E-FMAPs) by State, Selected Periods in FY 2008-FY 2014 104
TABLE 15.	Medicaid as a Share of States' Total Budgets and State-Funded Budgets, State FY 2011 106
TABLE 16.	National Health Expenditures by Type and Payer, 2011 108
TABLE 17.	Historical and Projected National Health Expenditures by Payer for Selected Years, 1970–2021 110
TABLE 18.	Characteristics of Non-Institutionalized Individuals by Source of Health Insurance, 2012 112
TABLE 19.	Income as a Percentage of the Federal Poverty Level (FPL) for Various Family Sizes, 2013 117

TABLE 20.	Supplemental Payments by State and Category, FY 2012 (millions)	118
TABLE 21.	Federal CHIP Allotments, FY 2012 and FY 2013 (millions)	122
TABLE 22.	Federal CHIPRA Bonus Payments (millions)	124

Overview

MACStats, a standing section in all Commission reports to the Congress, presents data and information on the Medicaid and CHIP programs that otherwise can be difficult to find and are spread across multiple sources. In this report, MACStats includes state-specific information about program enrollment, spending, eligibility levels, and federal medical assistance percentages (FMAPs). It also details benefits and permissable cost sharing under Medicaid, and the dollar amounts of common federal poverty levels (FPLs) used to determine eligibility for Medicaid and CHIP. In addition, it provides information that places these programs in the broader context of state budgets and national health expenditures.

Key points in this report include:

- Total Medicaid spending grew by only about 1 percent in fiscal year (FY) 2012, reaching $435.5 billion (Table 6). Total CHIP spending grew by less than 2 percent, reaching $12.2 billion (Table 8).

- Enrollment growth was also low. The number of individuals ever covered by Medicaid grew by less than 2 percent, from an estimated 71.7 million in FY 2011 to 72.6 million in FY 2012 (MACPAC communication with CMS Office of the Actuary; includes about one million individuals in the U.S. territories). CHIP enrollment grew from 8.2 million to 8.4 million (Table 3).

- Although there was little growth in total Medicaid spending in FY 2012, federal Medicaid spending decreased and state spending increased (Table 6). This is due in part to the expiration of a temporary increase in FMAPs that was in place through the third quarter of FY 2011 (Table 14).

- Medicaid as a share of state budgets varies depending on how it is measured (Table 15). Looking only at the state-funded portion of state budgets (that is, the portion financed from their own revenues), Medicaid's share was 13.4 percent in state fiscal year (SFY) 2011. After including federal funds in state budgets, a typical practice in other data sources, Medicaid's share was 23.7 percent in SFY 2011.

- The Medicaid and CHIP programs together accounted for 15.5 percent of national health expenditures in calendar year 2011, and their share is projected to reach 20 percent in the next decade (Tables 16 and 17).

- Few states changed income eligibility levels for Medicaid and CHIP in 2012 (Tables 9 through 11). This is due in part to a Patient Protection and Affordable Care Act (ACA, P.L. 111-148, as amended) provision that currently prohibits states from restricting their coverage, with an exception for adults above 133 percent FPL in states with a budget deficit.

TABLE 1. Medicaid and CHIP Enrollment as a Percentage of the U.S. Population, 2012

Medicaid and CHIP Enrollment	Administrative Data		Survey Data (NHIS)
	Ever enrolled during the year	Point in time	Point in time
Medicaid	71.6 million[1]	56.5 million[1]	Not available
CHIP	8.4 million	5.7 million	Not available
Totals for Medicaid and CHIP	80.0 million[1]	62.2 million[1]	50.5 million

U.S. Population	Census Bureau		Survey Data (NHIS)
	314.9 million	313.8 million	307.9 million, excluding active-duty military and individuals in institutions

Medicaid and CHIP Enrollment as a Percentage of U.S. Population			
	25.4%	19.8%	16.4%

Notes: Excludes U.S. territories. Medicaid and CHIP enrollment numbers obtained from administrative data include individuals who received limited benefits (e.g., emergency services only). Administrative data are estimates for FY 2012 (October 2011 through September 2012). By combining administrative totals from Medicaid and CHIP, some individuals may be double counted if they were enrolled in both programs during the year. Overcounting of enrollees in the administrative data may occur for other reasons (e.g., individuals may move and be enrolled in two states' Medicaid programs during the year). National Health Interview Survey (NHIS) data are based on interviews conducted between January and June 2012. NHIS excludes individuals in institutions (such as nursing homes) and active-duty military; in addition, surveys such as NHIS generally do not count limited benefits as Medicaid/CHIP coverage and respondents are known to underreport Medicaid and CHIP coverage. The Census Bureau number in the ever-enrolled column was the estimated U.S. resident population as of December 2012 (the month with the largest count); the number of residents ever living in the United States during the year is not available. The Census Bureau point-in-time number is the average estimated monthly number of U.S. residents for 2012.

For a more detailed discussion of why Medicaid and CHIP enrollment numbers can vary, see Table 1 in MACPAC's March 2012 MACStats. As indicated here, reasons include differences in the sources of data (e.g., administrative records versus survey interviews), the individuals included in the data (e.g., those receiving full versus limited benefits, those who are living in the community versus an institution such as a nursing home), and the enrollment period examined (e.g., ever during the year versus at a point in time).

1 Excludes about one million individuals in the U.S. territories.

Sources: MACPAC analysis based on the following: MACPAC communication with Office of the Actuary, Centers for Medicare & Medicaid Services; analysis of NHIS by the National Center for Health Statistics for MACPAC (see MACStats Table 18); CHIP Statistical Enrollment Data System (SEDS) data (see MACStats Table 3); and Bureau of the Census, *Population estimates, national totals: Vintage 2012.* http://www.census.gov/popest/data/national/totals/2012/index.html

MACStats

TABLE 2. Medicaid Enrollment by State and Selected Characteristics, FY 2010 (thousands)

State	Total	Basis of Eligibility[1]				All dual eligibles		Dual Eligible Status[2]			
								Dual eligibles with full benefits		Dual eligibles with limited benefits	
		Child	Adult	Disabled	Aged	Total	Age 65+	Total	Age 65+	Total	Age 65+
Total	**65,804**	**31,705**	**18,282**	**9,541**	**6,276**	**9,736**	**5,807**	**7,361**	**4,406**	**2,375**	**1,369**
Alabama	1,016	509	176	212	118	206	116	97	51	109	65
Alaska	126	70	31	17	9	14	8	14	7	0	0
Arizona	1,531	682	618	136	96	153	89	119	65	34	24
Arkansas	699	364	119	146	70	125	67	70	42	55	26
California	11,335	4,341	4,953	1,026	1,015	1,262	888	1,231	864	31	24
Colorado[3]	632	375	113	88	57	85	51	70	41	15	9
Connecticut	712	316	231	73	92	133	87	79	46	54	41
Delaware	225	92	94	25	14	26	14	12	7	14	7
District of Columbia	213	81	78	37	17	26	15	20	12	6	4
Florida	3,703	1,891	771	571	470	676	440	369	255	307	186
Georgia	1,870	1,107	304	285	173	272	160	138	81	135	79
Hawaii	261	108	101	27	25	35	24	31	21	4	2
Idaho[3]	223	137	30	39	17	32	16	22	11	10	5
Illinois	2,780	1,490	771	306	213	346	195	307	170	39	25
Indiana	1,174	648	262	174	90	166	81	106	57	60	24
Iowa	555	261	169	81	43	86	43	71	33	15	10
Kansas	394	223	57	77	38	68	35	48	26	20	9
Kentucky	907	434	145	233	96	185	94	110	57	75	37
Louisiana	1,177	612	229	222	114	191	111	109	62	81	50
Maine[3]	352	124	105	62	61	98	60	54	26	44	34
Maryland	952	454	277	145	76	120	68	80	45	40	23
Massachusetts	1,654	483	735	268	168	270	143	248	122	22	21
Michigan	2,257	1,175	587	353	142	275	131	240	113	35	18
Minnesota	936	444	265	131	97	143	77	129	69	14	9
Mississippi	772	400	116	167	89	158	89	83	49	74	40
Missouri[3]	1,033	545	190	203	94	181	90	164	81	17	9
Montana	133	76	22	23	13	24	13	16	9	8	4
Nebraska	250	144	45	38	23	41	21	38	19	3	2
Nevada	340	203	67	44	27	45	27	23	15	22	12

TABLE 2, Continued

State	Total	Basis of Eligibility[1]				All dual eligibles		Dual Eligible Status[2]					
		Child	Adult	Disabled	Aged			Dual eligibles with full benefits		Dual eligibles with limited benefits			
						Total	Age 65+	Total	Age 65+	Total	Age 65+		
New Hampshire	167	99	24	29	16	33	15	22	10	10	5		
New Jersey	1,026	567	132	175	151	210	139	183	120	27	19		
New Mexico	576	348	116	70	43	70	42	39	24	30	18		
New York	5,570	2,095	2,180	678	618	797	541	694	462	103	79		
North Carolina	1,876	982	391	319	184	324	180	253	139	71	41		
North Dakota	82	44	18	12	9	16	9	13	7	3	2		
Ohio	2,246	1,114	562	388	181	326	164	222	118	104	47		
Oklahoma	829	460	181	121	67	120	64	99	53	21	12		
Oregon	644	323	167	97	58	100	56	65	38	35	18		
Pennsylvania	2,417	1,079	502	594	241	415	226	348	185	68	41		
Rhode Island	205	92	43	41	29	42	24	36	21	6	4		
South Carolina	909	463	208	154	84	155	84	135	72	20	12		
South Dakota	131	77	22	19	13	22	13	14	8	8	4		
Tennessee	1,502	780	312	268	143	269	140	157	79	111	61		
Texas	4,844	3,098	665	635	447	666	436	421	282	245	154		
Utah	352	204	89	43	16	32	15	29	13	4	2		
Vermont	196	68	82	24	22	36	22	28	16	8	6		
Virginia	1,007	551	169	177	110	184	104	124	73	60	30		
Washington	1,353	759	291	206	97	172	93	129	74	43	20		
West Virginia	430	204	64	119	42	84	42	51	26	33	16		
Wisconsin[3]	1,139	452	392	152	143	213	139	195	128	18	12		
Wyoming	87	57	14	11	6	11	6	7	4	4	2		

Notes: Enrollment numbers generally include individuals ever enrolled in Medicaid-financed coverage during the year, even if for a single month; however, in the event individuals were also enrolled in CHIP-financed Medicaid coverage (i.e., Medicaid-expansion CHIP) during the year, they are excluded if their most recent enrollment month was in Medicaid-expansion CHIP. Numbers exclude individuals enrolled only in Medicaid-expansion CHIP during the year and enrollees in the territories.

Although state-level information is not yet available, the estimated number of individuals ever enrolled in Medicaid (excluding Medicaid-expansion CHIP) is 70.7 million for FY 2011 and 71.6 million for FY 2012. These FY 2011-FY 2012 figures exclude about one million enrollees in the territories (MACPAC communication with CMS Office of the Actuary, February 2013).

[1] Children and adults under age 65 who qualify for Medicaid on the basis of a disability are included in the disabled category. About 690,000 enrollees age 65 and older are identified in the data as disabled; given that disability is not an eligibility pathway for individuals age 65 and older, MACPAC recodes these enrollees as aged.

[2] Dual eligibles are enrolled in both Medicaid and Medicare; those with limited benefits only receive Medicaid assistance with Medicare premiums and cost sharing.

[3] FY 2010 data were unavailable (Colorado, Idaho, Missouri, Wisconsin) or did not reliably break out CHIP enrollees (Maine); for these states, FY 2009 data are shown instead.

Source: MACPAC analysis of Medicaid Statistical Information System (MSIS) annual person summary (APS) data from the Centers for Medicare & Medicaid Services as of February 2013

MACStats

TABLE 3. CHIP Enrollment by State, FY 2012

State	Program Type[1] (as of January 14, 2013)	Children			Adults			Total CHIP Enrollment
		Medicaid expansion	Separate CHIP	Total children enrolled	Parents	Pregnant women	Total adults enrolled	
Total	—	2,357,451	5,785,723	8,143,174	208,502	9,665	218,167	8,361,341
Alabama	Separate	—	112,972	112,972	—	—	—	112,972
Alaska	Medicaid Expansion	13,499	—	13,499	—	—	—	13,499
Arizona	Separate	—	35,679	35,679	—	—	—	35,679
Arkansas	Combination	110,905	3,151	114,056	10,238	—	10,238	124,294
California	Combination	439,892	1,344,140	1,784,032	—	—	—	1,784,032
Colorado	Separate	—	126,169	126,169	—	4,873	4,873	131,042
Connecticut	Separate	—	19,986	19,986	—	—	—	19,986
Delaware	Combination	88	12,762	12,850	—	—	—	12,850
District of Columbia	Medicaid Expansion	7,293	—	7,293	—	—	—	7,293
Florida	Combination	1,047	413,980	415,027	—	—	—	415,027
Georgia	Separate	—	258,425	258,425	—	—	—	258,425
Hawaii	Medicaid Expansion	33,764	—	33,764	—	—	—	33,764
Idaho	Combination	20,948	24,984	45,932	392	—	392	46,324
Illinois	Combination	169,021	178,883	347,904	—	—	—	347,904
Indiana	Combination	107,349	46,913	154,262	—	—	—	154,262
Iowa	Combination	21,252	59,202	80,454	—	—	—	80,454
Kansas	Separate	—	64,229	64,229	—	—	—	64,229
Kentucky	Combination	52,032	33,299	85,331	—	—	—	85,331
Louisiana	Combination	141,502	9,170	150,672	—	—	—	150,672
Maine	Combination	24,818	11,506	36,324	—	—	—	36,324
Maryland	Medicaid Expansion	131,898	—	131,898	—	—	—	131,898
Massachusetts	Combination	66,378	78,825	145,203	—	—	—	145,203
Michigan	Combination	15,670	65,759	81,429	—	—	—	81,429
Minnesota	Combination	126	3,978	4,104	—	—	—	4,104
Mississippi	Separate	—	93,257	93,257	—	—	—	93,257
Missouri	Combination	55,311	37,484	92,795	—	—	—	92,795
Montana	Combination	—	28,570	28,570	—	—	—	28,570
Nebraska	Combination	55,568	698	56,266	—	—	—	56,266

TABLE 3, Continued

State	Program Type[1] (as of January 14, 2013)	Children Medicaid expansion	Children Separate CHIP	Total children enrolled	Adults Parents	Adults Pregnant women	Total adults enrolled	Total CHIP Enrollment
Nevada[2]	Combination	–	29,854	29,854	–	–	–	29,854
New Hampshire	Medicaid Expansion	11,437	–	11,437	–	–	–	11,437
New Jersey	Combination	85,042	116,375	201,417	182,073	312	182,385	383,802
New Mexico	Medicaid Expansion	9,582	–	9,582	15,799	–	15,799	25,381
New York	Combination	–	547,671	547,671	–	–	–	547,671
North Carolina	Combination	59,066	200,912	259,978	–	–	–	259,978
North Dakota	Combination	2,292	5,371	7,663	–	–	–	7,663
Ohio[3]	Medicaid Expansion	280,650	–	280,650	–	–	–	280,650
Oklahoma	Combination	118,937	6,952	125,889	–	–	–	125,889
Oregon	Separate	–	121,962	121,962	–	–	–	121,962
Pennsylvania	Separate	–	271,642	271,642	–	–	–	271,642
Rhode Island	Combination	25,028	1,940	26,968	–	379	379	27,347
South Carolina	Medicaid Expansion	75,281	–	75,281	–	–	–	75,281
South Dakota	Combination	13,141	4,287	17,428	–	–	–	17,428
Tennessee	Combination	26,058	75,485	101,543	–	–	–	101,543
Texas	Separate	–	999,838	999,838	–	–	–	999,838
Utah	Separate	–	65,983	65,983	–	–	–	65,983
Vermont	Separate	–	7,570	7,570	–	–	–	7,570
Virginia	Combination	89,506	100,455	189,961	–	4,101	4,101	194,062
Washington	Separate	–	42,614	42,614	–	–	–	42,614
West Virginia	Separate	–	37,807	37,807	–	–	–	37,807
Wisconsin	Combination	93,070	76,269	169,339	–	–	–	169,339
Wyoming	Separate	–	8,715	8,715	–	–	–	8,715

Notes: Enrollment numbers generally include individuals ever enrolled during the year, even if for a single month; however, in the event individuals were in multiple categories during the year (for example, in Medicaid for the first half of the year but a separate CHIP program for the second half), the individual would only be counted in the most recent category. CHIP-funded coverage of childless adults was prohibited after December 31, 2009. New Jersey and Rhode Island cover targeted low-income pregnant women under a CHIP state plan option; all other CHIP-funded coverage of adults shown in the table was permitted through waivers.

1 Under CHIP, states have the option to use an expansion of Medicaid, a separate CHIP program, or a combination of both approaches.
2 Effective November 30, 2011, Nevada no longer covers pregnant women and parents with CHIP allotments due to funding constraints. The state did not provide enrollment data for CHIP-funded adults in FY 2012.
3 Ohio data are from FY 2011.

Sources: For numbers of children: MACPAC analysis of CHIP Statistical Enrollment Data System (SEDS) data from Centers for Medicare & Medicaid Services (CMS) as of February 22, 2013. For numbers of adults: CMS analysis for MACPAC of SEDS as of January 30, 2013. For CHIP program type: CMS, *Children's Health Insurance Program plan activity as of January 14, 2013*. http://www.medicaid.gov/CHIP/Downloads/CHIPMap-01-14-13.pdf

MACStats

TABLE 4. Child Enrollment in Medicaid-Financed Coverage by State, and CHIP-Financed Coverage by State and Family Income, FY 2011

State	Medicaid-Financed Children[1] All incomes	At or below 200% FPL Number	At or below 200% FPL Percentage	CHIP-Financed Children (Medicaid-expansion and Separate CHIP Coverage) From 200% through 250% FPL Number	From 200% through 250% FPL Percentage	Above 250% FPL Number	Above 250% FPL Percentage	CHIP-Financed children
Total	**36,116,614**	**7,212,683**	**88.6%**	**735,209**	**9.0%**	**195,282**	**2.4%**	**8,143,174**
Alabama[2]	866,094	91,507	81.0	15,128	13.4	6,337	5.6	112,972
Alaska	84,926	13,499	100.0	—	—	—	—	13,499
Arizona	931,500	35,679	100.0	—	—	—	—	35,679
Arkansas	407,464	114,056	100.0	—	—	—	—	114,056
California	4,540,732	1,509,506	84.6	260,778	14.6	13,748	0.8	1,784,032
Colorado	484,882	103,468	82.0	22,701	18.0	—	—	126,169
Connecticut	313,245	11,587	58.0	2,350	11.8	6,049	30.3	19,986
Delaware	89,544	12,850	100.0	—	—	—	—	12,850
District of Columbia	92,484	—	—	—	—	7293	100.0	7,293
Florida	2,055,426	415,027	100.0	—	—	—	—	415,027
Georgia	1,163,759	226,595	87.7	31,830	12.3	—	—	258,425
Hawaii	150,120	28,992	85.9	3,540	10.5	1,232	3.6	33,764
Idaho	208,877	45,932	100.0	—	—	—	—	45,932
Illinois	2,309,875	347,904	100.0	—	—	—	—	347,904
Indiana	699,362	139,972	90.7	14,290	9.3	—	—	154,262
Iowa	314,863	67,312	83.7	1,848	2.3	11,294	14.0	80,454
Kansas	229,947	59,668	92.9	3,804	5.9	757	1.2	64,229
Kentucky	483,119	85,331	100.0	—	—	—	—	85,331
Louisiana	672,626	145,628	96.7	5,044	3.3	—	—	150,672
Maine[3]	176,607	36,324	100.0	—	—	—	—	36,324
Maryland	475,033	39,250	29.8	87,373	66.2	5,275	4.0	131,898
Massachusetts	507,107	114,756	79.0	19,619	13.5	10,828	7.5	145,203
Michigan	1,204,841	81,429	100.0	—	—	—	—	81,429
Minnesota	499,857	3,907	95.2	53	1.3	144	3.5	4,104
Mississippi	457,446	93,257	100.0	—	—	—	—	93,257
Missouri	564,583	79,766	86.0	9,151	9.9	3,878	4.2	92,795
Montana	78,211	28,570	100.0	—	—	—	—	28,570
Nebraska	167,003	56,266	100.0	—	—	—	—	56,266
Nevada	246,929	28,228	94.6	1,235	4.1	391	1.3	29,854
New Hampshire	94,517	2,373	20.7	5,743	50.2	3,321	29.0	11,437

TABLE 4, Continued

State	Medicaid-Financed Children[1] All incomes	CHIP-Financed Children (Medicaid-expansion and Separate CHIP Coverage)						CHIP-Financed children
		At or below 200% FPL		From 200% through 250% FPL		Above 250% FPL		
		Number	Percentage	Number	Percentage	Number	Percentage	
New Jersey	659,379	153,511	76.2%	27,339	13.6%	20,567	10.2%	201,417
New Mexico	381,116	3,345	34.9	6,237	65.1	–	–	9,582
New York	2,209,544	382,831	69.9	92,151	16.8	72,689	13.3	547,671
North Carolina	1,151,887	253,815	97.6	3,819	1.5	2,344	0.9	259,978
North Dakota	50,037	7,663	100.0	–	–	–	–	7,663
Ohio[4]	1,214,287	280,650	100.0	–	–	–	–	280,650
Oklahoma	548,190	85,445	67.9	40,444	32.1	–	–	125,889
Oregon	399,823	110,918	90.9	7,711	6.3	3,333	2.7	121,962
Pennsylvania	1,310,974	231,392	85.2	28,700	10.6	11,550	4.3	271,642
Rhode Island	110,930	23,460	87.0	3,508	13.0	–	–	26,968
South Carolina	551,620	72,977	96.9	1,744	2.3	560	0.7	75,281
South Dakota[2]	47,387	17,428	100.0	–	–	–	–	17,428
Tennessee	761,274	89,226	87.9	12,317	12.1	–	–	101,543
Texas	3,518,832	999,838	100.0	–	–	–	–	999,838
Utah	281,386	65,983	100.0	–	–	–	–	65,983
Vermont	72,929	–	–	3,707	49.0	3,863	51.0	7,570
Virginia	637,131	189,961	100.0	–	–	–	–	189,961
Washington	775,909	12,880	30.2	19,905	46.7	9,829	23.1	42,614
West Virginia	260,672	34,874	92.2	2,933	7.8	–	–	37,807
Wisconsin	543,478	169,132	99.9	207	0.1	–	–	169,339
Wyoming	58,850	8,715	100.0	–	–	–	–	8,715

Notes: The definition in this table for Medicaid-financed children may differ from that used elsewhere in this report. This table includes children with and without disabilities; in tables using Medicaid eligibility categories, children qualifying on the basis of a disability are counted in the disabled category, not the child category.

In 2013, 200 percent of the federal poverty level (FPL) is $22,980 for an individual and $8,040 for each additional family member in the lower 48 states and the District of Columbia. For additional information, see MACStats Table 19.

Enrollment numbers generally include children ever enrolled during the year, even if for a single month; however, in the event children were in multiple categories during the year (for example, in Medicaid for the first half of the year but a separate CHIP program for the second half), the child would only be counted in the most recent category.

[1] MACPAC analysis of Statistical Enrollment Data System (SEDS) data found that 99.5 percent of Medicaid-financed children were at or below 200 percent FPL.

[2] Alabama data for Medicaid-financed children are from FY 2011.

[3] In SEDS, Delaware and South Dakota reported several thousand CHIP enrollees above 200 percent FPL, even though their CHIP programs are reported to only cover individuals up to 200 percent FPL; the numbers here were altered to put all of these enrollees at or below 200 percent FPL.

[4] Ohio data are from FY 2011.

Source: MACPAC analysis of CHIP Statistical Enrollment Data System (SEDS) data from the Centers for Medicare & Medicaid Services as of February 22, 2013.

MACStats

TABLE 5. Child Enrollment in Separate CHIP Programs by State and Managed Care Participation, FY 2012

State	Total[1]	Managed Care		Fee for Service		Primary Care Case Management	
		Number	Percentage	Number	Percentage	Number	Percentage
Total	**5,785,723**	**4,683,387**	**80.9%**	**892,513**	**15.4%**	**209,823**	**3.6%**
Alabama	112,972	—	—	112,972	100.0	—	—
Alaska	—	—	—	—	—	—	—
Arizona	35,679	34,228	95.9	1451	4.1	—	—
Arkansas	3,151	—	—	3,151	100.0	—	—
California	1,344,140	1,199,936	89.3	144,204	10.7	—	—
Colorado	126,169	126,169	100.0	—	—	—	—
Connecticut	19,986	—	—	19,986	100.0	—	—
Delaware	12,762	12,481	97.8	—	—	281	2.2
District of Columbia	—	—	—	—	—	—	—
Florida	413,980	400,458	96.7	5,016	1.2	8,506	2.1
Georgia	258,425	244,241	94.5	14,184	5.5	—	—
Hawaii	—	—	—	—	—	—	—
Idaho	24,984	—	—	—	—	24,984	100.0
Illinois	178,883	5,937	3.3	43,269	24.2	129,677	72.5
Indiana	46,913	41,575	88.6	5,338	11.4	—	—
Iowa	59,202	59,202	100.0	—	—	—	—
Kansas	64,229	64,180	99.9	49	0.1	—	—
Kentucky	33,299	32,748	98.3	188	0.6	363	1.1
Louisiana	9,170	244	2.7	8,713	95.0	213	2.3
Maine	11,506	—	—	3,795	33.0	7,711	67.0
Maryland	—	—	—	—	—	—	—
Massachusetts	78,825	28,374	36.0	28,712	36.4	21,739	27.6
Michigan	65,759	64,061	97.4	1,698	2.6	—	—
Minnesota	3,978	3,379	84.9	599	15.1	—	—
Mississippi	93,257	93,257	100.0	—	—	—	—
Missouri	37,484	14,748	39.3	22,736	60.7	—	—
Montana	28,570	—	—	28,570	100.0	—	—
Nebraska	698	—	—	698	100.0	—	—

TABLE 5, Continued

State	Total[1]	Managed Care		Fee for Service		Primary Care Case Management	
		Number	Percentage	Number	Percentage	Number	Percentage
Nevada	29,854	25,958	86.9%	3,896	13.1%	–	–
New Hampshire	–	–	–	–	–	–	–
New Jersey	116,375	113,570	97.6	2,805	2.4	–	–
New Mexico	–	–	–	–	–	–	–
New York	547,671	546,821	99.8	850	0.2	–	–
North Carolina	200,912	–	–	200,912	100.0	–	–
North Dakota	5,371	–	–	–	–	5,371	100.0%
Ohio	–	–	–	–	–	–	–
Oklahoma	6,952	–	–	6,952	100.0	–	–
Oregon	121,962	48,198	39.5	73,316	60.1	448	0.4
Pennsylvania	271,642	271,642	100.0	–	–	–	–
Rhode Island	1,940	1,940	100.0	–	–	–	–
South Carolina	–	–	–	–	–	–	–
South Dakota	4,287	–	–	1,373	32.0	2,914	68.0
Tennessee	75,485	–	–	75,485	100.0	–	–
Texas	999,838	999,838	100.0	–	–	–	–
Utah	65,983	65,983	100.0	–	–	–	–
Vermont	7,570	–	–	527	7.0	7,043	93.0
Virginia	100,455	87,346	87.0	12,715	12.7	394	0.4
Washington	42,614	25,871	60.7	16,564	38.9	179	0.4
West Virginia	37,807	–	–	37,807	100.0	–	–
Wisconsin	76,269	62,287	81.7	13,982	18.3	–	–
Wyoming	8,715	8,715	100.0	–	–	–	–

Notes: Enrollment numbers generally include children ever enrolled during the year, even if for a single month; however, in the event children were in multiple categories during the year the child would only be counted in the most recent category.

Categorizations of the types of delivery system are based on states' definitions and Statistical Enrollment Data System (SEDS) instructions to states. According to SEDS instructions, managed care includes arrangements under which the state contracts with a health maintenance or health insuring organization to provide a comprehensive set of services; enrollees choose a plan and a primary care provider (PCP) who will be responsible for managing their care. Under fee for service (FFS), providers submit claims to the state and are paid a specific amount for each service performed. Under primary care case management, providers are paid generally on a FFS basis, but PCPs are paid an additional flat monthly fee for each patient assigned to them for case management.

1 Because this table shows enrollment only in separate CHIP programs, these totals do not include child enrollment in Medicaid-expansion CHIP programs.

Source: MACPAC analysis of CHIP Statistical Enrollment Data System (SEDS) data from the Centers for Medicare & Medicaid Services as of February 22, 2013.

MACStats

TABLE 6. Medicaid Spending by State, Category, and Source of Funds, FY 2012 (millions)

State[1]	Benefits			State Program Administration			Total Medicaid		
	Total	Federal	State	Total	Federal	State	Total	Federal	State
Alabama	$4,981	$3,436	$1,545	$222	$153	$68	$5,202	$3,589	$1,613
Alaska	1,323	772	551	117	82	36	1,441	854	587
Arizona	7,903	5,452	2,451	264	187	77	8,167	5,639	2,528
Arkansas	4,105	2,908	1,197	257	166	91	4,362	3,074	1,288
California	48,884	25,011	23,873	4,387	2,511	1,876	53,271	27,522	25,749
Colorado	4,686	2,350	2,336	230	138	92	4,916	2,488	2,428
Connecticut	6,463	3,226	3,237	233	139	93	6,696	3,366	3,331
Delaware	1,484	806	678	88	60	29	1,573	866	707
District of Columbia	2,099	1,467	632	125	77	48	2,224	1,544	681
Florida	17,794	9,974	7,820	853	561	291	18,647	10,535	8,112
Georgia	8,299	5,488	2,811	496	331	165	8,795	5,819	2,976
Hawaii	1,451	727	724	61	36	25	1,512	763	749
Idaho	1,420	992	428	96	58	39	1,516	1,050	466
Illinois	13,216	6,648	6,569	779	457	322	13,995	7,105	6,891
Indiana	7,450	4,987	2,463	441	277	164	7,891	5,264	2,627
Iowa	3,417	2,081	1,336	157	109	48	3,574	2,190	1,384
Kansas	2,634	1,496	1,138	201	135	66	2,834	1,631	1,204
Kentucky	5,565	3,962	1,603	194	132	62	5,759	4,094	1,665
Louisiana	7,057	4,880	2,177	297	197	100	7,354	5,077	2,277
Maine	2,370	1,502	867	195	150	45	2,565	1,652	913
Maryland	7,564	3,791	3,774	340	207	133	7,904	3,998	3,907
Massachusetts	12,661	6,313	6,348	665	419	247	13,326	6,731	6,595
Michigan	12,377	8,210	4,168	564	351	213	12,941	8,560	4,381
Minnesota	8,661	4,363	4,298	343	180	162	9,004	4,544	4,460
Mississippi	4,432	3,300	1,133	186	138	48	4,618	3,438	1,181
Missouri	8,621	5,491	3,129	384	252	132	9,004	5,743	3,261
Montana	966	653	313	65	43	23	1,031	695	336
Nebraska	1,676	952	724	116	72	44	1,792	1,024	768
Nevada	1,731	979	751	101	66	36	1,832	1,045	787
New Hampshire	1,174	592	583	76	45	31	1,251	637	614
New Jersey	10,263	5,136	5,127	708	431	277	10,971	5,567	5,404
New Mexico	3,420	2,410	1,010	184	131	53	3,604	2,541	1,063
New York	51,477	25,795	25,683	1,596	974	622	53,074	26,769	26,305
North Carolina	12,074	7,890	4,184	802	528	274	12,876	8,418	4,458
North Dakota	732	409	323	56	36	19	788	446	342
Ohio	16,242	10,404	5,838	585	364	221	16,826	10,768	6,058
Oklahoma	4,398	2,842	1,556	246	163	83	4,644	3,005	1,639

TABLE 6, Continued

State[1]	Benefits Total	Benefits Federal	Benefits State	State Program Administration Total	State Program Administration Federal	State Program Administration State	Total Medicaid Total	Total Medicaid Federal	Total Medicaid State
Oregon	$4,543	$2,875	$1,668	$379	$228	$151	$4,922	$3,103	$1,819
Pennsylvania	20,216	11,123	9,093	934	561	374	21,150	11,684	9,466
Rhode Island	1,842	966	875	103	65	37	1,944	1,032	912
South Carolina	4,611	3,242	1,369	204	138	66	4,815	3,381	1,434
South Dakota	740	465	275	45	27	18	786	492	293
Tennessee	8,751	5,827	2,924	499	309	190	9,250	6,135	3,115
Texas	27,523	16,075	11,448	1,410	861	550	28,934	16,936	11,998
Utah	1,871	1,329	541	133	81	52	2,003	1,410	593
Vermont	1,333	766	567	29	26	4	1,362	792	570
Virginia	6,807	3,412	3,395	283	167	116	7,089	3,579	3,511
Washington	7,453	3,763	3,690	667	408	259	8,120	4,171	3,949
West Virginia	2,772	2,012	760	158	109	50	2,931	2,121	810
Wisconsin	6,978	4,257	2,722	486	310	176	7,464	4,566	2,898
Wyoming	518	263	255	48	32	15	566	296	270
Subtotal (States)	**$407,028**	**$234,072**	**$172,956**	**$22,090**	**$13,676**	**$8,414**	**$429,118**	**$247,748**	**$181,370**
American Samoa	29	16	13	0	0	0	29	16	13
Guam	48	26	21	2	1	1	50	27	22
Northern Mariana Islands	25	14	11	0	0	0	25	14	11
Puerto Rico	1,614	888	726	54	27	26	1,667	915	752
Virgin Islands	10	6	4	1	0	0	10	6	4
Subtotal (States & Territories)	**$408,752**	**$235,021**	**$173,731**	**$22,147**	**$13,706**	**$8,442**	**$430,899**	**$248,726**	**$182,173**
State Medicaid Fraud Control Units (MFCUs)	—	—	—	288	216	72	288	216	72
Medicaid survey and certification of nursing and intermediate care facilities	—	—	—	304	228	76	304	228	76
Vaccines for Children (VFC) program	—	—	—	—	—	—	4,009	4,009	—
Total	**$408,752**	**$235,021**	**$173,731**	**$22,739**	**$14,150**	**$8,590**	**$435,500**[2]	**$253,179**[2]	**$182,321**

Notes: Total federal spending shown here ($253.179 billion) will differ from total federal outlays shown in FY 2013 budget documents due to slight differences in the timing of data for the states and the treatment of certain adjustments. Benefits and Administration columns do not sum to Total Medicaid due to the inclusion of VFC in Total Medicaid. Federal spending in the territories is capped; however, they report their total spending regardless of whether they have reached their caps. As a result, federal spending shown here may exceed the amounts actually paid to the territories. State shares for MFCUs and survey and certification are MACPAC estimates based on 75 percent federal match. State-level estimates for these items are available but are not shown here. VFC is authorized in the Medicaid statute but is operated as a separate program; 100 percent federal funding finances the purchase of vaccines for children who are enrolled in Medicaid, uninsured, or privately insured without vaccine coverage. Spending on administration is only for state programs; federal oversight spending is not included. Zeroes indicate amounts less than $0.5 million that round to zero. Dashes indicate amounts that are true zeroes.

1 Not all states have certified their CMS-64 Financial Management Report (FMR) submissions as of February 25, 2013. Idaho's 3rd quarter submission is not certified; Alabama and California's 4th quarter submissions are not certified. Figures presented in this table may change once all states have finalized and certified their expenditure data.

2 Amount exceeds the sum of Benefits and State Program Administration columns due to the inclusion of VFC.

Sources: MACPAC analysis of CMS-64 Financial Management Report (FMR) net expenditure data as of February 2013 for the states and territories; Centers for Medicare & Medicaid Services (CMS), *Fiscal year 2013 justification of estimates for Appropriations Committees*, Baltimore, MD: CMS, for MFCUs, survey and certification, VFC

MACStats

TABLE 7. Total Medicaid Benefit Spending by State and Category, FY 2012 (millions)

State[1]	Total	Fee for Service									Managed Care and Premium Assistance	Medicare Premiums and Coinsurance	Collections
		Hospital	Physician	Dental	Other practitioner	Clinic and health center	Other acute	Drugs	Institutional LTSS	Home and community-based LTSS			
Alabama	$4,981	$1,896	$331	$86	$38	$82	$492	$305	$999	$445	$102	$250	-$46
Alaska	1,323	296	103	63	20	198	95	31	163	356	0	22	-25
Arizona	7,903	896	32	4	5	114	239	5	64	6	6,336	205	-2
Arkansas	4,105	978	283	75	18	186	702	153	989	467	17	291	-55
California	48,884	11,449	882	449	24	2,556	6,507	987	5,800	7,566	11,699	2,248	-1,281
Colorado	4,686	1,599	295	104	—	121	321	144	667	810	568	95	-38
Connecticut	6,463	1,739	212	156	86	270	296	331	1,709	1,265	368	328	-296
Delaware	1,484	65	17	33	1	41	83	66	149	120	878	33	-0
District of Columbia	2,099	412	46	20	2	115	126	63	304	393	597	34	-12
Florida	17,794	4,936	1,081	189	45	232	1,410	575	3,314	1,569	3,312	1,245	-113
Georgia	8,299	2,130	376	43	33	166	563	245	1,339	895	2,439	295	-227
Hawaii	1,451	75	5	29	-2	30	15	2	10	103	1,169	57	-42
Idaho	1,420	387	91	0	10	108	189	55	245	277	50	40	-31
Illinois	13,216	4,875	663	204	117	325	1,269	785	2,602	1,454	719	380	-176
Indiana	7,450	1,590	224	164	10	319	302	352	1,777	837	1,751	161	-36
Iowa	3,417	810	177	59	76	68	302	121	898	631	217	138	-78
Kansas	2,634	415	97	38	6	28	122	71	576	567	664	83	-34
Kentucky	5,565	616	111	14	9	195	369	-39	1,071	581	2,563	212	-137
Louisiana	7,057	2,115	411	121	—	146	385	789	1,421	795	916	259	-302
Maine	2,370	482	106	32	50	217	366	68	392	425	6	270	-43
Maryland	7,564	997	79	120	17	53	867	226	1,271	987	2,843	227	-122
Massachusetts	12,661	2,204	288	201	22	319	1,740	118	1,913	2,003	3,710	407	-265
Michigan	12,377	1,628	353	82	7	227	771	278	1,896	930	5,901	389	-83
Minnesota	8,661	635	190	28	198	49	485	104	1,034	2,163	3,836	172	-232
Mississippi	4,432	1,628	290	9	29	80	450	194	1,097	255	234	201	-34
Missouri	8,621	3,017	21	15	14	462	552	613	1,556	1,062	1,094	307	-106
Montana	966	253	48	22	15	14	178	39	188	179	7	31	-7
Nebraska	1,676	278	59	31	8	72	82	85	399	318	287	103	-46
Nevada	1,731	498	91	26	11	15	168	65	253	164	338	112	-8
New Hampshire	1,174	180	55	21	8	84	140	37	355	283	—	24	-12
New Jersey	10,263	1,743	45	14	4	194	622	17	2,876	1,023	3,515	335	-126
New Mexico	3,420	513	48	14	43	31	50	14	32	312	2,296	78	-10
New York	51,477	10,146	332	239	243	1,421	2,642	-872	11,527	9,854	16,484	1,278	-1,828
North Carolina	12,074	4,413	1,068	329	28	256	1,582	477	1,769	1,228	687	417	-208
North Dakota	732	123	50	10	7	10	42	23	303	161	4	11	-12
Ohio	16,242	2,210	296	48	22	160	677	-1	3,779	2,332	6,448	383	-110
Oklahoma	4,398	1,581	452	124	32	371	322	294	681	499	153	133	-244

TABLE 7, Continued

State[1]	Total	Fee for Service								Managed Care and Premium Assistance	Medicare Premiums and Coinsurance	Collections
		Hospital	Physician	Dental	Other practitioner	Clinic and health center	Other acute	Drugs	Institutional LTSS	Home and community-based LTSS			
Oregon	$4,543	$366	$27	$0	$25	$51	$309	$66	$352	$1,095	$2,144	$151	-$44
Pennsylvania	20,216	2,071	213	77	9	138	480	191	4,623	2,974	9,068	550	-178
Rhode Island	1,842	342	12	11	1	22	532	-0	339	2	535	40	-14
South Carolina	4,611	1,121	191	85	25	228	318	115	801	462	1,329	172	-237
South Dakota	740	185	56	15	2	84	56	25	168	129	2	27	-9
Tennessee	8,751	1,351	26	172	1	37	200	386	245	512	5,533	335	-47
Texas	27,523	5,939	1,184	688	448	79	2,427	282	3,783	2,456	9,983	1,016	-762
Utah	1,871	598	115	40	4	15	124	105	253	223	392	33	-33
Vermont	1,333	44	2	0	0	1	1,285	-113	116	7	6	6	-20
Virginia	6,807	1,055	194	136	37	56	909	72	1,263	1,159	1,804	223	-100
Washington	7,453	1,347	192	137	58	385	432	172	875	1,525	2,129	308	-107
West Virginia	2,772	480	143	55	14	30	238	120	701	553	341	114	-17
Wisconsin	6,978	658	45	42	22	291	642	293	1,100	698	3,048	255	-118
Wyoming	518	117	50	13	24	18	25	17	123	132	0	8	-10
Subtotal	**$407,028**	**$85,479**	**$11,755**	**$4,687**	**$1,926**	**$10,771**	**$33,498**	**$8,554**	**$70,160**	**$55,241**	**$118,515**	**$14,493**	**-$8,125**
American Samoa	29	7	4	0	—	2	19	0	0	—	—	—	-4
Guam	48	8	4	0	0	0	26	8	0	—	—	1	—
N. Mariana Islands	25	16	—	1	—	3	1	2	—	1	—	0	—
Puerto Rico	1,614	—	—	—	—	—	31	—	—	—	1,582	—	—
Virgin Islands	10	7	0	0	—	1	0	1	0	—	—	0	—
Total	**$408,752**	**$85,517**	**$11,763**	**$4,689**	**$1,926**	**$10,777**	**$33,576**	**$8,565**	**$70,161**	**$55,242**	**$120,098**	**$14,495**	**-$8,129**
Percent of Total, Exclusive of Collections	—	20.5%	2.8%	1.1%	0.5%	2.6%	8.1%	2.1%	16.8%	13.3%	28.8%	3.5%	—

Notes: Includes federal and state funds. Service category definitions and spending amounts shown here may differ from other CMS data sources such as the Medicaid Statistical Information System (MSIS). Readers should note that MACPAC refined its methodology for classifying services in its June 2012 report. Major changes included shifting mental health facility out of the hospital category and into the institutional long-term services and supports (LTSS) category and shifting rehabilitation, private duty nursing, targeted case management, and hospice out of the home and community-based LTSS category and into the other acute category. An additional change to the March 2013 classification includes shifting drug rebates for managed care organizations from the drug category to the managed care and premium assistance category. ICF-ID is intermediate care facility for the intellectually disabled; LTSS is long-term services and supports. Hospital includes inpatient, outpatient, critical access hospital, and emergency hospital services, as well as related disproportionate share hospital (DSH) payments. Other practitioner includes nurse midwife, nurse practitioner, and other. Clinic and health center includes non-hospital outpatient clinic, rural health clinic, federally qualified health center, and freestanding birth center. Other acute includes lab/X-ray; sterilizations; abortions; Early and Periodic Screening, Diagnostic, and Treatment (EPSDT) screenings; emergency services for unauthorized aliens; non-emergency transportation; physical, occupational, speech, and hearing therapy; prosthetics, dentures, and eyeglasses; diagnostic screening and preventive services; school-based services; health home with chronic conditions; tobacco cessation for pregnant women; private duty nursing; case management (excluding primary care case management); rehabilitative services; hospice; and other care not otherwise categorized. Drugs are net of rebates. Institutional LTSS includes nursing facility, ICF-ID, and mental health facility. Home and community-based (HCB) services include home health, HCB waiver and state plan services, and personal care. Managed care and premium assistance includes comprehensive and limited-benefit managed care plans, primary care case management (PCCM), employer-sponsored premium assistance programs, Programs of All-inclusive Care for the Elderly (PACE), and rebates for drugs provided by managed care plans; comprehensive plans account for about 90 percent of spending in the managed care category. Collections include third-party liability, estate, and other recoveries. Zeroes indicate amounts less than $0.5 million that round to zero. Dashes indicate amounts that are true zeroes.

1 Not all states have certified their CMS-64 Financial Management Report (FMR) submissions as of February 25, 2013. Idaho's 3rd quarter submission is not certified; Alabama and California's 4th quarter submissions are not certified. Figures presented in this table may change once all states have finalized and certified their expenditure data.

Source: MACPAC analysis of CMS-64 Financial Management Report (FMR) net expenditure data as of February 2013

MACStats

TABLE 8. CHIP Spending by State, FY 2012 (millions)

State	Total CHIP[1]		Benefits						State Program Administration			2105(g) Spending[1]
			Medicaid-expansion CHIP programs			Separate CHIP programs and adult coverage waivers						
	Total	Federal	State	Total	Federal	State	Total	Federal	State	Total	Federal	State	Federal
Alabama	$200.8	$156.7	$44.1	—	—	—	$192.2	$149.9	$42.2	$8.6	$6.7	$1.9	—
Alaska	30.4	19.8	10.6	$29.2	$19.0	$10.2	—	—	—	1.2	0.8	0.4	—
Arizona	31.6	24.4	7.2	—	—	—	30.0	23.2	6.8	1.6	1.3	0.4	—
Arkansas	124.8	99.2	25.6	95.7	76.1	19.6	23.4	18.6	4.8	5.7	4.5	1.2	—
California	1,918.3	1,246.8	671.5	405.3	263.5	141.9	1,436.2	933.5	502.7	76.8	49.9	26.9	—
Colorado	194.2	126.3	68.0	—	—	—	194.8	126.6	68.2	-0.6	-0.4	-0.2	—
Connecticut	25.4	39.8	-14.4	—	—	—	23.0	15.1	7.9	2.4	1.6	0.8	$23.1
Delaware	22.3	15.1	7.1	-0.7	-0.5	-0.2	21.2	14.4	6.8	1.8	1.2	0.6	—
District of Columbia	17.6	13.9	3.7	17.2	13.6	3.6	—	—	—	0.3	0.3	0.1	—
Florida	499.1	345.4	153.7	3.7	2.5	1.1	445.6	308.4	137.2	49.8	34.5	15.3	—
Georgia	355.8	271.6	84.2	—	—	—	324.4	247.6	76.8	31.3	23.9	7.4	—
Hawaii	38.5	24.8	13.8	35.5	22.8	12.7	—	—	—	3.0	2.0	1.1	—
Idaho	43.7	34.6	9.1	12.8	10.1	2.6	29.4	23.2	6.1	1.5	1.2	0.3	—
Illinois	407.6	265.1	142.5	135.7	88.2	47.5	250.6	163.0	87.6	21.3	13.8	7.4	—
Indiana	181.3	139.4	41.9	122.8	94.4	28.4	53.2	40.9	12.3	5.4	4.1	1.2	—
Iowa	122.7	89.0	33.8	27.0	19.5	7.4	88.3	64.0	24.3	7.5	5.5	2.1	—
Kansas	76.3	53.3	23.0	—	—	—	69.6	48.6	21.0	6.7	4.7	2.0	—
Kentucky	178.2	142.3	35.9	110.7	88.4	22.3	64.5	51.5	13.0	3.0	2.4	0.6	—
Louisiana	226.9	165.1	61.8	192.4	140.0	52.4	20.4	14.8	5.5	14.2	10.3	3.9	—
Maine	40.7	30.3	10.4	24.3	18.0	6.2	13.2	9.8	3.4	3.3	2.4	0.8	—
Maryland	237.5	154.4	83.1	225.7	146.7	79.0	—	—	—	11.8	7.7	4.1	—
Massachusetts	489.7	318.3	171.4	225.7	146.7	79.0	215.1	139.8	75.3	49.0	31.8	17.1	—
Michigan	66.2	52.7	13.5	-18.2	-11.6	-6.5	80.8	61.6	19.1	3.6	2.7	0.8	—
Minnesota	19.6	30.9	-11.2	0.1	0.1	0.0	19.1	12.4	6.6	0.5	0.3	0.2	18.1
Mississippi	207.6	170.2	37.4	—	—	—	207.3	169.9	37.4	0.3	0.2	0.0	—
Missouri	158.9	118.3	40.7	110.9	82.5	28.4	45.0	33.5	11.5	3.0	2.3	0.8	—
Montana	74.9	57.1	17.8	17.3	13.2	4.1	52.5	40.0	12.4	5.2	4.0	1.2	—
Nebraska	58.5	40.8	17.8	54.9	38.2	16.7	—	—	—	3.6	2.5	1.1	—
Nevada	43.9	30.3	13.6	7.5	5.0	2.5	34.3	23.8	10.5	2.1	1.5	0.6	—
New Hampshire	20.1	17.5	2.6	3.6	2.3	1.2	15.8	10.3	5.5	0.8	0.5	0.3	4.4
New Jersey	947.2	615.9	331.3	179.8	116.9	62.9	672.6	437.4	235.2	94.7	61.6	33.1	—
New Mexico	151.6	119.1	32.5	67.2	52.8	14.4	83.7	65.7	17.9	0.8	0.6	0.2	—

TABLE 8, Continued

State	Total CHIP[1]			Benefits						State Program Administration			2105(g) Spending[1]
				Medicaid-expansion CHIP programs			Separate CHIP programs and adult coverage waivers						
	Total	Federal	State	Total	Federal	State	Total	Federal	State	Total	Federal	State	Federal
New York	$858.0	$557.8	$300.2	$152.4	$99.1	$53.3	$695.4	$452.0	$243.3	$10.2	$6.6	$3.6	—
North Carolina	385.7	292.0	93.7	64.9	49.1	15.8	301.7	228.4	73.3	19.1	14.5	4.6	—
North Dakota	24.0	16.5	7.5	9.9	6.8	3.1	12.9	8.9	4.0	1.2	0.8	0.4	—
Ohio	431.7	323.3	108.4	426.8	319.6	107.2	—	—	—	4.9	3.7	1.2	—
Oklahoma	146.1	109.2	36.9	133.3	99.6	33.7	9.8	7.4	2.5	3.0	2.2	0.8	—
Oregon	187.0	138.4	48.5	—	—	—	174.1	128.9	45.2	12.8	9.5	3.3	—
Pennsylvania	429.0	294.1	134.9	—	—	—	421.6	289.0	132.6	7.5	5.1	2.3	—
Rhode Island	57.2	38.0	19.1	41.5	27.6	13.9	14.5	9.7	4.9	1.2	0.8	0.4	—
South Carolina	119.2	94.4	24.8	109.3	86.5	22.8	—	—	—	10.0	7.9	2.1	—
South Dakota	26.2	18.7	7.5	19.0	13.5	5.5	6.7	4.8	1.9	0.5	0.3	0.1	—
Tennessee	252.0	192.6	59.3	46.9	35.9	11.0	186.6	142.7	43.9	18.4	14.1	4.3	—
Texas	1,200.7	849.1	351.6	39.3	27.8	11.5	1,096.0	775.0	320.9	65.4	46.3	19.2	—
Utah	74.8	59.6	15.2	—	—	—	70.9	56.5	14.4	3.9	3.1	0.8	—
Vermont	9.2	12.5	-3.4	—	—	—	8.4	5.9	2.5	0.7	0.5	0.2	—
Virginia	276.0	179.4	96.6	116.3	75.6	40.7	149.8	97.3	52.4	9.9	6.5	3.5	$6.1
Washington	71.7	93.0	-21.3	13.3	8.6	4.6	56.1	36.5	19.6	2.3	1.5	0.8	—
West Virginia	57.5	46.4	11.0	—	—	—	54.1	43.7	10.4	3.3	2.7	0.6	46.4
Wisconsin	131.8	99.1	32.7	54.5	39.3	15.2	70.6	51.1	19.5	6.8	4.9	1.9	—
Wyoming	15.9	10.4	5.5	—	—	—	15.2	9.9	5.3	0.7	0.4	0.2	3.8
Subtotal	**$11,965.7**	**$8,452.7**	**$3,513.1**	**$3,313.2**	**$2,337.4**	**$975.8**	**$8,050.3**	**$5,595.5**	**$2,454.8**	**$602.3**	**$418.0**	**$184.3**	**$101.8**
American Samoa	1.5	1.3	0.3	1.5	1.3	0.3	—	—	—	—	—	—	—
Guam	6.1	4.4	1.7	6.1	4.4	1.7	—	—	—	—	—	—	—
N. Mariana Islands	1.0	0.9	0.1	1.0	0.9	0.1	—	—	—	—	—	—	—
Puerto Rico	186.3	127.6	58.7	186.3	127.6	58.7	—	—	—	—	—	—	—
Virgin Islands	15.9	10.4	5.5	—	—	—	—	—	—	—	—	—	—
Total	**$12,160.7**	**$8,586.8**	**$3,573.9**	**$3,508.1**	**$2,471.5**	**$1,036.6**	**$8,050.3**	**$5,595.5**	**$2,454.8**	**$602.3**	**$418.0**	**$184.3**	**$101.8**

Notes: Components may not add to total due to rounding. As shown in Table 3, some states have waivers under Section 1115 of the Social Security Act that use CHIP funds to provide coverage for adults (pregnant women and parents). Federal CHIP spending on administration is generally limited to 10 percent of a state's total federal CHIP spending for the year. States with a Medicaid-expansion CHIP program may elect to receive reimbursement for administrative spending from Medicaid rather than CHIP funds; Medicaid funds are not shown in this table. Zeroes indicate amounts less than $0.5 million that round to zero. Dashes indicate amounts that are true zeroes.

1 Section 2105(g) of the Social Security Act permits 11 qualifying states to use CHIP funds to pay the difference between the regular Medicaid matching rate and the enhanced CHIP matching rate for Medicaid-enrolled, Medicaid-financed children whose family income exceeds 133 percent of the federal poverty level. Since there is no state share of CHIP spending for these children (because their state share is financed entirely under Medicaid), some states (Connecticut, Minnesota, Vermont, and Washington) are shown in this table as having negative state CHIP spending.

Source: MACPAC analysis of Medicaid and CHIP Budget Expenditure System (MBES/CBES) data from CMS as of December 2012

TABLE 9. Medicaid and CHIP Income Eligibility Levels as a Percentage of the Federal Poverty Level for Children and Pregnant Women by State, February 2013

Medicaid coverage of children under age 19 with incomes below states' eligibility levels in effect as of March 31, 1997, continues to be financed by Medicaid. Any expansion above those levels—through expansions of Medicaid or through separate CHIP programs—is generally financed by CHIP. Adult pregnant women can receive Medicaid- or CHIP-funded services through regular state plan eligibility pathways or Section 1115 waivers; in addition, the unborn children of pregnant women may receive CHIP-funded coverage under a state plan option. Deemed newborns are infants up to age 1 who are deemed eligible for Medicaid or CHIP—with no separate application or eligibility determination required—if their mother was enrolled at the time of their birth.

	Medicaid Coverage						CHIP Program Type[2] (as of January 14, 2013)	Separate CHIP Coverage		Medicaid/CHIP Coverage
	Infants under age 1		Age 1 through 5		Age 6 through 18			Birth through age 18	Unborn children	Pregnant women and deemed newborns[3]
State	Medicaid funded[1]	CHIP funded[1]	Medicaid funded[1]	CHIP funded[1]	Medicaid funded[1]	CHIP funded[1]				
Alabama	133%	–	133%	–	100%	–	Separate	300%	–	133%
Alaska	133	175%	133	175%	100	175%	Medicaid Expansion	–	–	175
Arizona	140	–	133	–	100	–	Separate	200[4]	–	150
Arkansas[5]	133	200	133	200	100	200	Combination	–	200%	200
California[6]	200	250	133	250	100	250	Combination	250/300[7]	300	200
Colorado	133	–	133	–	100	–	Separate	250	–	133/200[8]
Connecticut	185	–	185	–	185	–	Separate	300	–	250
Delaware	133	200	133	–	100	–	Combination	200	–	200
District of Columbia	185	300	133	300	100	300	Medicaid Expansion	–	–	300
Florida	185	200	133	–	100	–	Combination	200	–	185
Georgia	185	–	133	–	100	–	Separate	235	–	200
Hawaii	185	300	133	300	100	300	Medicaid Expansion	–	–	185
Idaho	133	–	133	–	100	133	Combination	185	–	133
Illinois	133	–	133	–	100	133	Combination	200	200	200
Indiana	150	–	133	150	100	150	Combination	250[9]	–	200
Iowa	185	300	133	–	100	133	Combination	300	–	300
Kansas	150	–	133	–	100	–	Separate	232	–	150
Kentucky	185	–	133	150	100	150	Combination	200	–	185
Louisiana	133	200	133	200	100	200	Combination	250	200	200
Maine	185	–	133	150	125	150	Combination	200	–	200
Maryland	185	300	185	300	185	300	Medicaid Expansion	–	–	250
Massachusetts	185	200	133	150	114	150	Combination	300	200[10]	200
Michigan	185	–	133	150	100	150	Combination	200	185	185

TABLE 9, Continued

	Medicaid Coverage						CHIP Program Type[2] (as of January 14, 2013)	Separate CHIP Coverage		Medicaid/CHIP Coverage
	Infants under age 1		Age 1 through 5		Age 6 through 18			Birth through age 18	Unborn children	Pregnant women and deemed newborns[3]
State	Medicaid funded[1]	CHIP funded[1]	Medicaid funded[1]	CHIP funded[1]	Medicaid funded[1]	CHIP funded[1]				
Minnesota	275%	280%[11]	275%	–	275%	–	Combination	–	275%	275%
Mississippi	185	–	133	–	100	–	Separate	200%	–	185
Missouri	185	–	133	150%	100	150%	Combination	300	–	185
Montana	133	–	133	–	100	133	Combination	250	–	150
Nebraska	150	200	133	200	100	200	Combination	–	185	185
Nevada	133	–	133	–	100	–	Combination	200	–	133/185[12]
New Hampshire	185	300	185	300	185	300	Medicaid Expansion	–	–	185
New Jersey	185	–	133	–	100	133	Combination	350	–	185/200[13]
New Mexico	185	235	185	235	185	235	Medicaid Expansion	–	–	235
New York	185	–	133	–	100	133	Combination	400	–	200
North Carolina	185	200	133	200	100	–	Combination	200	–	185
North Dakota[14]	133	133	133	133	100	100	Combination	160	–	133
Ohio[15]	133	200	133	200	100	200	Medicaid Expansion	–	–	200
Oklahoma[16]	150	185	133	185	100	185	Combination	200	185	185
Oregon	133	–	133	–	100	–	Separate	300	185	185
Pennsylvania	185	–	133	–	100	–	Separate	300	–	185
Rhode Island[17]	250	–	250	–	100	250	Combination	–	250	185/250[18]
South Carolina	185	200	133	200	100	200	Medicaid Expansion	–	–	185
South Dakota	133	140	133	140	100	140	Combination	200	–	133
Tennessee[19]	185	200	133	200	100	200	Combination	250	250	185
Texas	185	–	133	–	100	–	Separate	200	200	185
Utah	133	–	133	–	100	–	Separate	200	–	133
Vermont	225	–	225	–	225	–	Separate	300	–	200
Virginia	133	–	133	–	100	133	Combination	200	–	133/200[20]
Washington	200	–	200	–	200	–	Separate	300	185	185
West Virginia	150	–	133	–	100	–	Separate	300	–	150
Wisconsin	185	–	185	–	100	150	Combination	300	300	300
Wyoming	133	–	133	–	100	–	Separate	200	–	133

TABLE 9, Continued

Notes: In 2013, 100 percent of the federal poverty level (FPL) in the lower 48 states and the District of Columbia is $11,490 for an individual and $4,020 for each additional family member. For additional information, see MACStats Table 19. Eligibility levels shown here apply to countable income; for some eligibility pathways, states may use various income disregards that result in different amounts of countable income. Some states achieve the eligibility levels listed by applying block disregards that exclude a specified amount of income. Some numbers may differ in practice because of the operation of an income disregard that has not been taken into account.

1 The eligibility levels listed under Medicaid funded are generally the Medicaid eligibility thresholds as of March 31, 1997. The eligibility levels listed under CHIP funded are the income levels to which Medicaid has expanded with CHIP funding since its creation in 1997. In 1997, many states had different eligibility levels for children age 6 through 13 and age 14 through 18; in such cases, this table shows the 1997 levels for children age 6 through 13.

2 Under CHIP, states have the option to use an expansion of Medicaid, a separate CHIP program, or a combination of both approaches.

3 Pregnant women can be covered with Medicaid or CHIP funding. When pregnant women are covered under CHIP, coverage can be through a state plan option for targeted low-income pregnant women or through a Section 1115 waiver. Values in this column are for Medicaid-covered pregnant women, except where noted.

4 Arizona's CHIP program has been closed to new enrollment since January 1, 2010.

5 Arkansas was approved to expand its separate CHIP program to 250 percent FPL effective January 1, 2011 but this has not been implemented. Arkansas' separate CHIP enrollment is only for unborn children.

6 In California, children through age 18 who are no longer eligible for Medicaid and who are converting to the separate CHIP program are covered for one month under the Medicaid expansion program as a bridge while their CHIP enrollment is processed.

7 California's county program expanded eligibility to 300 percent FPL under its separate CHIP program in four counties (three of the four counties have implemented this provision), with all other counties at 250 percent FPL. During 2013, California is transitioning to a Medicaid-expansion CHIP program.

8 Colorado covers pregnant women up to 133 percent FPL under Medicaid and from 134 through 200 percent FPL under CHIP through a Section 1115 waiver.

9 Indiana's increase of the income threshold from 250 to 300 percent FPL was approved November 18, 2009, but the state has not yet implemented the expansion.

10 Massachusetts has been approved to provide coverage of unborn children up to 225 percent FPL, but the state has only implemented up to 200 percent FPL.

11 In Minnesota, infants are defined as being under age 2. Only infants are eligible for the Medicaid-expansion CHIP program.

12 Nevada covers pregnant women up to 133 percent FPL under Medicaid and from 134 through 185 percent FPL under CHIP through a Section 1115 waiver. Nevada's Medicaid-expansion CHIP program consists of children who became eligible for Medicaid when the state eliminated the Medicaid asset test.

13 New Jersey covers pregnant women up to 185 percent FPL under Medicaid and from 186 through 200 percent FPL under CHIP through a state plan option for targeted low-income pregnant women.

14 North Dakota's Medicaid-expansion CHIP program consists of children who became eligible for Medicaid when the state eliminated the Medicaid asset tests.

15 Ohio has been approved to increase the income threshold to 300 percent FPL, but the state has not yet implemented the expansion.

16 Oklahoma covers certain children with physical or mental disabilities, referred to as Katie Beckett children, from 0 through 200 percent FPL as a Medicaid expansion in all age groups (under a program created by the Tax Equity and Fiscal Responsibility Act of 1982). Oklahoma has been approved to increase the income threshold of its separate CHIP program to 300 percent FPL, but has implemented the expansion up to 200 percent FPL.

17 In Rhode Island, the age ranges are 1 through 7 and 8 through 18. The state has increased the Medicaid expansion CHIP program income threshold to 300 percent FPL, but it has not been implemented. The state's separate CHIP program covers unborn children only.

18 Rhode Island covers pregnant women up to 185 percent FPL under Medicaid and from 186 through 250 percent FPL under CHIP through a state plan option for targeted low-income pregnant women.

19 Tennessee covers children as a Medicaid expansion group with CHIP funding, called TennCare Standard, but this Section 1115 waiver is currently capped except for children who "rollover" from traditional Medicaid. This includes children with a family income above Medicaid income levels, but at or below 200 percent FPL, who are losing TennCare Medicaid eligibility.

20 Virginia covers pregnant women up to 133 percent FPL under Medicaid and from 134 through 200 percent FPL under CHIP through a Section 1115 waiver.

Source: MACPAC communication with CMS and analysis of state websites

MACStats

MACStats

TABLE 10. Medicaid Income Eligibility Levels as a Percentage of the Federal Poverty Level for Non-Aged, Non-Disabled, Non-Pregnant Adults by State, January 2013

States are required to provide Medicaid coverage for parents (and their dependent children), at a minimum, at their 1996 Aid to Families with Dependent Children eligibility levels. Under regular Medicaid state plan rules, states may opt to cover additional parents (via Section 1931 of the Social Security Act) and other adults under age 65 who are not pregnant, not eligible for Medicare, and have incomes below 133 percent of the federal poverty level (via Section 1902(a)(10)(A)(i)(VIII) of the Social Security Act). States may also provide coverage under Section 1115 waivers, which allow them to operate their Medicaid programs without regard to certain statutory requirements. As noted throughout this table, the covered benefits under these waivers may be more limited than those provided under regular state plan rules and may not be available to all individuals at the income levels shown. In addition, regardless of whether coverage is provided under a waiver, jobless and working individuals may qualify at different income levels due to disregards of certain amounts of earned income. States may use additional disregards (such as child care expenses) that are not accounted for here.

| | Parents of Dependent Children[1] | | | | Other Adults[1] | | | |
| | Jobless | | Working | | Jobless | | Working | |
State	Medicaid benefits[2]	More limited coverage	Medicaid benefits[2]	More limited coverage	Medicaid benefits[2]	More limited coverage	Medicaid benefits[2]	More limited coverage
Alabama	10%	–	23%	–	–	–	–	–
Alaska	74	–	78	–	–	–	–	–
Arizona[3]	100	–	106	–	100% (closed)	–	100% (closed)	–
Arkansas[4]	13	200%	16	200%	–	–	–	200%
California[5]	100	–	106	206	–	200%	–	210
Colorado[6]	100	–	106	–	10 (closed)	–	20 (closed)	–
Connecticut	185	–	191	–	55	–	70	–
Delaware	100	–	120	–	100	–	110	–
District of Columbia	200	–	206	–	200	–	211	–
Florida	19	–	56	–	–	–	–	–
Georgia	27	–	48	–	–	–	–	–
Hawaii[7]	133	–	133	–	133	–	133	–
Idaho[8]	20	–	37	185	–	–	–	185
Illinois[9,10]	133	–	139	–	–	–	–	–
Indiana[11]	18	200	24	206	–	200 (closed)	–	210 (closed)
Iowa[12]	27	200	80	250	–	200	–	250
Kansas	25	–	31	–	–	–	–	–
Kentucky	33	–	57	–	–	–	–	–
Louisiana[13]	11	–	24	–	–	–	–	–

TABLE 10, Continued

State	Parents of Dependent Children[1]				Other Adults[1]			
	Jobless		Working		Jobless		Working	
	Medicaid benefits[2]	More limited coverage	Medicaid benefits[2]	More limited coverage	Medicaid benefits[2]	More limited coverage	Medicaid benefits[2]	More limited coverage
Maine[14]	200%	—	200%	—	—	100% (closed)	—	100% (closed)
Maryland[15]	116	—	122	—	—	116	—	128
Massachusetts[16]	133	300%	133	300%	—	300	—	300
Michigan[17]	37	—	64	—	—	35 (closed)	—	45 (closed)
Minnesota[18]	215	275	215	275	75%	200	75%	200
Mississippi	23	—	29	—	—	—	—	—
Missouri[19]	18	—	35	—	—	—	—	—
Montana	31	—	54	—	—	—	—	—
Nebraska	47	—	58	—	—	—	—	—
Nevada	24	—	84	—	—	—	—	—
New Hampshire	38	—	47	—	—	—	—	—
New Jersey[20]	200 (closed >133)	200 (closed)	200 (closed >133)	—	—	23	—	23
New Mexico[21]	28	—	85	408 (closed)	—	200 (closed)	—	414 (closed)
New York[22]	150	—	150	—	100	—	100	—
North Carolina	34	—	47	—	—	—	—	—
North Dakota	33	—	57	—	—	—	—	—
Ohio	90	—	96	—	—	—	—	—
Oklahoma[23]	36	—	51	200	—	—	—	200
Oregon[24]	30	100 (closed)	39	201 (closed)	—	100 (closed)	—	201 (closed)
Pennsylvania	25	—	58	—	—	—	—	—
Rhode Island[25]	175	—	181	—	—	—	—	—
South Carolina	50	—	89	—	—	—	—	—
South Dakota	50	—	50	—	—	—	—	—
Tennessee	67	—	122	—	—	—	—	—
Texas	12	—	25	—	—	—	—	—
Utah[26]	37	150 (closed)	42	200	150	150 (closed)	—	200
Vermont[27]	185	300	191	331	160	300	160	353
Virginia	25	—	30	—	—	—	—	—
Washington[28]	35	133 (closed)	71	200 (closed)	—	133 (closed)	—	200 (closed)
West Virginia	16	—	31	—	—	—	—	—
Wisconsin[29]	200	—	200	—	—	200 (closed)	—	200 (closed)
Wyoming	37	—	50	—	—	—	—	—

TABLE 10, Continued

Notes: In 2013, the federal poverty level (100 percent FPL) is $11,490 for an individual and $4,020 for each additional family member in the lower 48 states and the District of Columbia. For additional information, see MACStats Table 19.

1 The table reflects income eligibility levels at time of application. It also takes earning disregards, when applicable, into account when determining income thresholds for working adults. For parents, computations are based on a family of three with one earner; for other adults, computations are based on an individual. In some cases, earnings disregards may be time limited and only applied for the first few months of coverage; in these cases, eligibility limits for most enrollees would be lower than the levels that appear in this table. States may use additional disregards in determining eligibility. In some states, the income eligibility guidelines vary by region; in this situation, the income guideline in the most populous region is used. "Closed" indicates that the state was not enrolling new adults eligible for coverage into a program at any point between January 1, 2012 and January 1, 2013.

2 This column does not differentiate by coverage authority, only by the scope of the benefit package. States may expand coverage to parents and other adults through Section 1115 waivers that provide full Medicaid benefits or more limited coverage.

3 Arizona froze enrollment in its waiver coverage for childless adults on July 8, 2011.

4 In Arkansas, adults up to 200 percent FPL are eligible for more limited subsidized coverage under the ARHealthNetworks waiver program; individuals must have income below the eligibility threshold and work for a qualifying, participating employer.

5 California extends coverage for adults through two programs: the Medicaid Coverage Expansion (MCE) up to 133 percent FPL and the Health Care Coverage Initiative (HCCI) between 133 and 200 percent FPL. While both coverage options offer more limited benefits than full Medicaid, the MCE benefit package is more comprehensive. Fifty out of 58 counties are participating in MCE; five counties are participating in HCCI.

6 Colorado extended Medicaid coverage to a limited number of adults (10,000) with income up to 10 percent FPL through a waiver as of May 2012.

7 Hawaii reduced coverage for parents and other adults to 133 percent FPL in 2012.

8 Idaho provides premium assistance to adults up to 185 percent FPL under a waiver; individuals must have income below the eligibility threshold and work for a qualified small employer.

9 Illinois reduced Medicaid eligibility for Section 1931 parents from 200 to 133 percent FPL in 2012.

10 In Illinois, adults with income up to 133 percent FPL who reside in Cook County are eligible for Medicaid as of November 2012.

11 In Indiana, adults up to 200 percent FPL are eligible for limited coverage under the Healthy Indiana waiver program; enrollment is closed for childless adults.

12 In Iowa, adults up to 200 percent FPL are eligible for more limited coverage under the IowaCare waiver program.

13 In Louisiana, adults with income up to 200 percent FPL who reside in the Greater New Orleans area are eligible for more limited coverage through the Greater New Orleans Community Health Connection Section 1115 Waiver.

14 Maine received approval of a State Plan Amendment to reduce eligibility for Section 1931 parents from 200 to 133 percent FPL in January 2013. The state plans to implement the cuts on March 1, 2013. Childless adults up to 100 percent FPL are eligible for more limited coverage under the MaineCare waiver program; enrollment is closed.

15 In Maryland, childless adults are eligible for primary care services under the Primary Adult Care waiver program.

16 In Massachusetts, childless adults who are long-term unemployed or clients of the Department of Mental Health with income below 100 percent FPL can receive more limited benefits under the MassHealth waiver program through MassHealth Basic or Essential. Additionally, adults up to 300 percent FPL are eligible for more limited subsidized coverage under the Commonwealth Care waiver program.

17 In Michigan, childless adults are eligible for more limited coverage under the Adult Benefit Waiver program; enrollment is closed.

18 In Minnesota, parents up to 215 percent FPL receive full Medicaid benefits with the exception of some optional services (e.g., non-emergency transportation, private duty nursing, personal care, orthodontic services, targeted case management) and institutionally based long-term care services. Parents above 215 percent FPL and childless adults receive a more limited benefit package that has a $10,000 annual limit on inpatient hospital care. Minnesota decreased eligibility for childless adults in its Section 1115 and state-funded coverage from 250 to 200 percent FPL in 2012.

19 In Missouri, adults with income up to 200 percent FPL who reside in the St. Louis area are eligible for more limited coverage through the Gateway to Better Health Section 1115 waiver.

20 In New Jersey, parents up to 200 percent FPL are covered under the FamilyCare waiver program. Waiver enrollment closed in 2010 for parents who do not qualify for Medicaid using an enhanced-income disregard. In April 2011, New Jersey obtained a waiver to expand coverage to childless adults who had previously been covered through the state's general assistance program. For those who are unemployable, the limit is $210 per individual; for those who are employable, the limit is $140 per individual.

21 In New Mexico, adults up to 200 percent FPL are eligible for more limited subsidized coverage under the State Coverage Insurance waiver program. Individuals must have income below the eligibility threshold and work for a participating employer; if they do not work for a participating employer, they can obtain coverage by paying both the employer and employee share of premium costs; enrollment is closed.

22 In New York, childless adults up to 78 percent FPL are eligible for the Medicaid (Home Relief) waiver program, and parents up to 150 percent FPL and childless adults up to 100 percent FPL are eligible for the Family Health Plus waiver program.

23 In Oklahoma, adults up to 200 percent FPL are eligible for more limited subsidized coverage under the Insure Oklahoma waiver program. Individuals must have income below the eligibility threshold and also work for a small employer or be self-employed, unemployed and seeking work, working disabled, a full-time college student, or the spouse of a qualified worker.

24 In Oregon, adults up to 100 percent FPL are eligible for more limited coverage under the Oregon Health Plan (OHP) Standard waiver program; enrollment in OHP Standard is closed. The state provides premium assistance to adults up to 201 percent FPL under its Family Health Insurance Assistance Program (FHIAP) waiver program; enrollment in FHIAP is open to children only.

25 In Rhode Island, parents up to 175 percent FPL are covered under the RIteCare and RIteShare waiver programs.

26 In Utah, adults up to 150 percent FPL are eligible for coverage of primary care services under the Primary Care Network waiver program; enrollment is closed. The state also provides premium assistance for employer-sponsored coverage to working adults under the Utah Premium Partnership (UPP) Health Insurance waiver program. Eligibility in UPP increased from 150 to 200 percent in October 2012.

TABLE 10, Continued

27 In Vermont, Section 1931 coverage is available up to 77 percent FPL in urban areas and 73 percent FPL in rural areas; parents up to 185 percent FPL and childless adults up to 150 percent FPL are eligible for the Vermont Health Access Plan waiver program. Additionally, the state offers more limited subsidized coverage to adults up to 300 percent FPL under its Catamount Health waiver program.

28 In Washington, adults up to 133 percent FPL are eligible for more limited coverage under the state's Basic Health waiver, enrollment is closed.

29 In Wisconsin, childless adults up to 200 percent FPL are eligible for more limited coverage under the BadgerCare Plus Core Plan waiver program; enrollment for childless adults is closed. In 2012, the state changed its crowd-out policy for parents and adults; if health insurance costs 9.5 percent or less of income, they are excluded from coverage.

Source: M. Heberlein et al., *Getting into gear for 2014: Findings from a 50-state survey of eligibility, enrollment, renewal, and cost-sharing policies in Medicaid and CHIP, 2012-2013*, Washington, DC: Kaiser Commission on Medicaid and the Uninsured, January 2013. http://www.kff.org/medicaid/upload/8401.pdf

TABLE 11. Medicaid Income Eligibility Levels as a Percentage of the Federal Poverty Level for Individuals Age 65 and Older and Persons with Disabilities by State, 2012

In most states, enrollment in the Supplemental Security Income (SSI) program for individuals age 65 and older and persons with disabilities automatically qualifies them for Medicaid. However, 11 209(b) states may use more restrictive criteria than SSI when determining Medicaid eligibility. In all states, additional people with low incomes or high medical expenses may be covered, at the state's option, through poverty level, medically needy, special income level, and other eligibility pathways.

State	State Eligibility Type[1]	SSI Recipients	209(b) Eligibility Levels	Poverty Level[2]	Medically Needy[3]	Special Income Level[4]
Alabama	1634	75%	–	–	–	225%
Alaska[5]	SSI Criteria	60	–	–	–	225
Arizona	1634	75	–	100%	–	225
Arkansas	1634	75	–	80 (Aged only)	12%	225
California	1634	75	–	100	64	100
Colorado	1634	75	–	–	–	225
Connecticut	209(b)	–	66%	–	66	225
Delaware	1634	75	–	–	–	188
District of Columbia	1634	75	–	100	64	225
Florida	1634	75	–	88	19	225
Georgia	1634	75	–	–	34	225
Hawaii	209(b)	–	100	100	45	–
Idaho	SSI Criteria	75	–	–	–	225
Illinois	209(b)	–	100	–	100	–
Indiana	209(b)	–	75	–	–	225
Iowa	1634	75	–	–	52	225
Kansas	SSI Criteria	75	–	–	51	225
Kentucky	1634	75	–	–	23	225
Louisiana	1634	75	–	75	10	225
Maine	1634	75	–	100	34	225
Maryland	1634	75	–	–	38	225
Massachusetts	1634	75	–	100(Aged)/133(Disabled)	58	225
Michigan	1634	75	–	100	44	225
Minnesota	209(b)	–	53	100	75	225
Mississippi	1634	75	–	–	–	225
Missouri	209(b)	–	85	85	–	133
Montana	1634	75	–	–	67	–
Nebraska	SSI Criteria	75	–	100	42	–
Nevada	SSI Criteria	75	–	–	–	225

TABLE 11, Continued

State	State Eligibility Type[1]	SSI Recipients	209(b) Eligibility Levels	Poverty Level[2]	Medically Needy[3]	Special Income Level[4]
New Hampshire	209(b)	–	76%	–	63%	225%
New Jersey	1634	75%	–	100%	39	225
New Mexico	1634	75	–	–	–	225
New York	1634	75	–	85	85	–
North Carolina	1634	75	–	100	26	–
North Dakota	209(b)	–	83	–	83	–
Ohio	209(b)	–	64	–	–	225
Oklahoma	209(b)	–	79	100	–	225
Oregon	SSI Criteria	75	–	–	–	225
Pennsylvania	1634	75	–	100	46	225
Rhode Island	1634	75	–	100	90	225
South Carolina	1634	75	–	100	–	225
South Dakota	1634	75	–	–	–	225
Tennessee	1634	75	–	–	26[6]	225
Texas	1634	75	–	–	–	225
Utah	SSI Criteria	75	–	100	100	225
Vermont	1634	75	–	–	110	225
Virginia	209(b)	–	80	80	48	225
Washington	1634	75	–	–	75	225
West Virginia	1634	75	–	–	21	225
Wisconsin	1634	75	–	–	64	225
Wyoming	1634	75	–	–	–	225

Notes: In 2013, the federal poverty level (100 percent FPL) is $11,490 for an individual and $4,020 for each additional family member in the lower 48 states and the District of Columbia. For additional information, see MACStats Table 19. Eligibility levels shown here apply to countable income; for some eligibility pathways, states may use various income disregards that result in different amounts of countable income. The eligibility levels listed in this table are for individuals; the eligibility levels for couples differ for certain categories.

[1] Both Section 1634 and SSI-criteria states use SSI criteria for Medicaid eligibility. In Section 1634 states, the federal eligibility determination process for SSI automatically qualifies an individual for Medicaid; in SSI-criteria states, individuals must submit information to the state for a separate eligibility determination. Section 209(b) states may use eligibility criteria more restrictive than the SSI program but may not use more restrictive criteria than those in effect in the state on January 1, 1972; they must also allow individuals with higher incomes to spend down to the 209(b) income level shown here by deducting incurred medical expenses from the amount of income that is counted for Medicaid eligibility purposes.

[2] Under the poverty level option, states may choose to provide Medicaid coverage to persons who are aged or disabled and whose income is above the SSI or 209(b) level, but at or below the FPL.

[3] Under the medically needy option, individuals with higher incomes can spend down to the medically needy income level shown here by deducting incurred medical expenses from the amount of income that is counted for Medicaid eligibility purposes. Five states (Connecticut, Louisiana, Michigan, Vermont, and Virginia) have a medically needy income standard that varies by location. In these instances, the highest income standard is listed.

[4] Under the special income level option, states have the option to provide Medicaid benefits to people who require at least 30 days of nursing home or other institutional care and have incomes up to 300 percent of the SSI benefit rate (which is about 225 percent FPL). The income standard listed in this column may be for institutional services, home and community-based waiver services, or both.

[5] The dollar amount that equals the upper income eligibility level for SSI does not vary by state; however, the dollar amount that equals the FPL is higher in Alaska (see MACStats Table 19), resulting in a lower percentage.

[6] Category not currently open to new enrollees.

Sources: MACPAC analysis of eligibility information from state websites and Medicaid state plans as of February 2013

TABLE 12. Mandatory and Optional Medicaid Benefits

Although mandatory and optional Medicaid benefits are listed in federal statute, the breadth of coverage (i.e., amount, duration, and scope) varies by state. When designing a benefit, states may elect to place no limits on a benefit, or they may choose to limit a benefit by requiring prior approval of the service, restricting the place of service, or employing utilization controls or dollar caps. For example, while most states cover dental services, and some even cover annual dental exams, others limit this benefit to trauma care or emergency treatment for pain relief and infection, require that services be provided in a specific setting (such as an emergency room), require that certain services have prior approval, or place dollar caps on the total amount of services an enrollee can receive each year. The result is that the same benefit can be designed and implemented in a number of different ways across states.

The table on the following page lists mandatory and optional Medicaid benefits that are described in federal statute or regulations. No single source of information currently provides an up-to-date, comprehensive picture of the optional benefits covered by states and the circumstances under which a given benefit is covered. Readers may instead refer to a number of sources including, for example:

- Centers for Medicare & Medicaid Services, U.S. Department of Health and Human Services, *State Medicaid benefits matrix*, December 2010 and January 2011. https://www.cms.gov/Medicare/Health-Plans/SpecialNeedsPlans/Downloads/StateMedicaidBenefitsMatrix042011.zip
- Kaiser Family Foundation, *Medicaid benefits: Online database*. http://medicaidbenefits.kff.org/
- Kaiser Commission on Medicaid and the Uninsured, *Coverage of preventive services for adults in Medicaid*, September 2012. http://www.kff.org/medicaid/upload/8359.pdf
- Substance Abuse and Mental Health Services Administration, U.S. Department of Health and Human Services, *State profiles of mental health and substance abuse services in Medicaid*, January 2005. http://store.samhsa.gov/product/State-Profiles-of-Mental-Health-and-Substance-Abuse-Services-in-Medicaid/NMH05-0202

TABLE 12, Continued

Mandatory Medicaid Benefits

- Inpatient hospital services
- Outpatient hospital services
- Physician services
- Early and Periodic Screening, Diagnostic, and Treatment (EPSDT) services for individuals under age 21 (screening, vision, dental, and hearing services and any medically necessary service listed in the Medicaid statute, including optional services that are not otherwise covered by a state)
- Family planning services and supplies
- Federally qualified health center services
- Freestanding birth center services
- Home health services
- Laboratory and x-ray services
- Nursing facility services (for ages 21 and over)
- Nurse midwife services (to the extent authorized to practice under state law or regulation)
- Certified pediatric or family nurse practitioner services (to the extent authorized to practice under state law or regulation)
- Rural heath clinic services
- Tobacco cessation counseling and pharmacotherapy for pregnant women
- Non-emergency transportation to medical care[1]

Optional Medicaid Benefits

- Prescribed drugs
- Intermediate care facility services for individuals with intellectual disabilities
- Clinic services
- Occupational therapy services
- Optometry services
- Physical therapy services
- Targeted case management services
- Prosthetic devices
- Hospice services
- Inpatient psychiatric services for individuals under age 21
- Dental services
- Eyeglasses
- Speech, hearing, and language disorder services
- Inpatient hospital and nursing facility services for individuals age 65 or older in institutions for mental diseases
- Emergency hospital services in a hospital not meeting certain Medicare or Medicaid requirements[2]
- Dentures
- Personal care services
- Private duty nursing services
- Program of All-inclusive Care for the Elderly (PACE) services
- Chiropractic services
- Critical access hospital services
- Respiratory care for ventilator-dependent individuals
- Primary care case management services
- Services furnished in a religious nonmedical health care institution
- Tuberculosis-related services
- Home and community-based services
- Health homes for enrollees with chronic conditions
- Other licensed practitioners' services
- Other diagnostic, screening, preventive, and rehabilitative services

Notes:

1 Federal regulations require states to provide transportation services; they may do so as an administrative function or as part of the Medicaid benefits package.

2 Federal regulations define these services as being those that are necessary to prevent the death or serious impairment of the health of the recipient and, because of the threat to life, necessitates the use of the most accessible hospital available that is equipped to furnish the services, even if the hospital does not currently meet Medicare's participation requirements or the definition of inpatient or outpatient hospital services under Medicaid rules.

Source: Centers for Medicare & Medicaid Services, *Medicaid benefits*, as of February 2013. http://www.medicaid.gov/Medicaid-CHIP-Program-Information/By-Topics/Benefits/Medicaid-Benefits.html

MAC Stats

TABLE 13. Maximum Allowable Medicaid Premiums and Cost Sharing, FY 2013

	At or Below 100% FPL	From 100% through 150% FPL	Above 150% FPL
Exempt Populations	Exempt populations for most types of cost sharing include children under age 18, pregnant women, beneficiaries receiving hospice care, beneficiaries in nursing facilities and intermediate care facilities for the intellectually disabled, certain enrollees in hospitals and other medical institutions, and American Indians who are furnished a Medicaid item or service through an Indian Health Service provider or through a contract health service referral.		
Exempt Services	Emergency services and family planning services and supplies are excluded from cost sharing.		
Cap for Alternative Cost Sharing[1]	Alternative cost sharing not permitted. Nominal amounts always apply.	When a state imposes alternative cost sharing above nominal amounts, the total amount of premiums and cost sharing may not exceed 5% of a family's monthly or quarterly income.	
Premium	Not permitted	Not permitted	Up to $19 a month for some populations, no limit for others (subject to 5% cap)
Non-Institutional Services	Deductible: Up to $2.65 Copayment: Up to $3.90	Deductible: Up to $2.65 Copayment: Up to 10% of the payment made by the Medicaid agency for the service	Deductible: Up to $2.65 Copayment: Up to 20% of the payment made by the Medicaid agency for the service
Institutional Services	Per admission, the deductible, coinsurance, or copayment made by the Medicaid agency for the first day of care.	Per admission, the deductible, coinsurance, or copayment may not exceed 50% of the payment made by the Medicaid agency for the first day of care or 10% of the cost of the item or service.	Per admission, the deductible, coinsurance, or copayment may not exceed 50% of the payment made by the Medicaid agency for the first day of care or 20% of the cost of the item or service.
Non-Emergency Care Provided in Emergency Room	Up to $3.90	Up to $7.80	No limit (subject to 5% cap)
Prescribed Drugs	Preferred and non-preferred copayment: Up to $3.90	Preferred and non-preferred copayment: Up to $3.90	Preferred copayment: Up to $3.90 Non-preferred: Up to 20% of the cost of the drug

Notes: In 2013, the federal poverty level (100 percent FPL) is $11,490 for an individual and $4,020 for each additional family member in the lower 48 states and the District of Columbia. For additional information, see MACStats Table 19.

This table contains FY 2013 numbers, where nominal is defined as being $2.65 for a monthly deductible or up to $3.90 for a copayment. The table does not reflect amounts that states may have implemented under a Section 1115 waiver.

[1] As first authorized in the Deficit Reduction Act of 2005 (P.L. 109-171), alternative cost sharing allows states to target cost sharing above nominal levels to specific groups of enrollees, provided their family income is above 100 percent FPL.

Sources: Sections 1916 and 1916A of the Social Security Act; 42 CFR 447; Centers for Medicare & Medicaid Services, *Cost sharing*, as of February 2013. http://www.medicaid.gov/Medicaid-CHIP-Program-Information/By-Topics/Cost-Sharing/Cost-Sharing-Out-of-Pocket-Costs.html

MACStats

TABLE 14. Federal Medical Assistance Percentages (FMAPs) and Enhanced FMAPs (E-FMAPs) by State, Selected Periods in FY 2008-FY 2014

State	FY 2008	FMAPs for Medicaid					E-FMAPs for CHIP			
		First quarter of FY 2011 (includes temporary increase)[1]	Fourth quarter of FY 2011 (regular formula level)	FY 2012	FY 2013	FY 2014[2]	FY 2012	FY 2013	FY 2014	
Alabama	67.62%	78.00%	68.54%	68.62%	68.53%	68.12%	78.03%	77.97%	77.68%	
Alaska	52.48	62.46	50.00	50.00	50.00	50.00	65.00	65.00	65.00	
Arizona	66.20	75.93	65.85	67.30	65.68	67.23	77.11	75.98	77.06	
Arkansas	72.94	81.18	71.37	70.71	70.17	70.10	79.50	79.12	79.07	
California	50.00	61.59	50.00	50.00	50.00	50.00	65.00	65.00	65.00	
Colorado	50.00	61.59	50.00	50.00	50.00	50.00	65.00	65.00	65.00	
Connecticut	50.00	61.59	50.00	50.00	50.00	50.00	65.00	65.00	65.00	
Delaware	50.00	64.38	53.15	54.17	55.67	55.31	67.92	68.97	68.72	
District of Columbia	70.00	79.29	70.00	70.00	70.00	70.00	79.00	79.00	79.00	
Florida	56.83	67.64	55.45	56.04	58.08	58.79	69.23	70.66	71.15	
Georgia	63.10	75.16	65.33	66.16	65.56	65.93	76.31	75.89	76.15	
Hawaii	56.50	67.35	51.79	50.48	51.86	51.85	65.34	66.30	66.30	
Idaho	69.87	79.18	68.85	70.23	71.00	71.64	79.16	79.70	80.15	
Illinois	50.00	61.88	50.20	50.00	50.00	50.00	65.00	65.00	65.00	
Indiana	62.69	76.21	66.52	66.96	67.16	66.92	76.87	77.01	76.84	
Iowa	61.73	72.55	62.63	60.71	59.59	57.93	72.50	71.71	70.55	
Kansas	59.43	69.68	59.05	56.91	56.51	56.91	69.84	69.56	69.84	
Kentucky	69.78	80.61	71.49	71.18	70.55	69.83	79.83	79.39	78.88	
Louisiana[3]	72.47	81.48	68.04	69.78	65.51	62.11	72.76	72.87	72.69	
Maine	63.31	74.86	63.80	63.27	62.57	61.55	74.29	73.80	73.09	
Maryland	50.00	61.59	50.00	50.00	50.00	50.00	65.00	65.00	65.00	
Massachusetts	50.00	61.59	50.00	50.00	50.00	50.00	65.00	65.00	65.00	
Michigan	58.10	75.57	65.79	66.14	66.39	66.32	76.30	76.47	76.42	
Minnesota	50.00	61.59	50.00	50.00	50.00	50.00	65.00	65.00	65.00	
Mississippi	76.29	84.86	74.73	74.18	73.43	73.05	81.93	81.40	81.14	
Missouri	62.42	74.43	63.29	63.45	61.37	62.03	74.42	72.96	73.42	
Montana	68.53	77.99	66.81	66.11	66.00	66.33	76.28	76.20	76.43	
Nebraska	58.02	68.76	58.44	56.64	55.76	54.74	69.65	69.03	68.32	
Nevada	52.64	63.93	51.61	56.20	59.74	63.10	69.34	71.82	74.17	
New Hampshire	50.00	61.59	50.00	50.00	50.00	50.00	65.00	65.00	65.00	
New Jersey	50.00	61.59	50.00	50.00	50.00	50.00	65.00	65.00	65.00	
New Mexico	71.04	80.49	69.78	69.36	69.07	69.20	78.55	78.35	78.44	
New York	50.00	61.59	50.00	50.00	50.00	50.00	65.00	65.00	65.00	
North Carolina	64.05	74.98	64.71	65.28	65.51	65.78	75.70	75.86	76.05	
North Dakota	63.75	69.95	60.35	55.40	52.27	50.00	68.78	66.59	65.00	

TABLE 14, Continued

State	FY 2008	FMAPs for Medicaid — First quarter of FY 2011 (includes temporary increase)[1]	Fourth quarter of FY 2011 (regular formula level)	FY 2012	FY 2013	FY 2014[2]	E-FMAPs for CHIP — FY 2012	FY 2013	FY 2014
Ohio	60.79%	73.71%	63.69%	64.15%	63.58%	63.02%	74.91%	74.51%	74.11%
Oklahoma	67.10	76.73	64.94	63.88	64.00	64.02	74.72	74.80	74.81
Oregon	60.86	72.97	62.85	62.91	62.44	63.14	74.04	73.71	74.20
Pennsylvania	54.08	66.58	55.64	55.07	54.28	53.52	68.55	68.00	67.46
Rhode Island	52.51	64.22	52.97	52.12	51.26	50.11	66.48	65.88	65.08
South Carolina	69.79	79.58	70.04	70.24	70.43	70.57	79.17	79.30	79.40
South Dakota	60.03	70.80	61.25	59.13	56.19	53.54	71.39	69.33	67.48
Tennessee	63.71	75.62	65.85	66.36	66.13	65.29	76.45	76.29	75.70
Texas[4]	60.56	70.94	60.56	58.22	59.30	58.69	70.75	71.51	71.08
Utah	71.63	80.78	71.13	70.99	69.61	70.34	79.69	78.73	79.24
Vermont	59.03	69.96	58.71	57.58	56.04	55.11	70.31	69.23	68.58
Virginia	50.00	61.59	50.00	50.00	50.00	50.00	65.00	65.00	65.00
Washington	51.52	62.94	50.00	50.00	50.00	50.00	65.00	65.00	65.00
West Virginia	74.25	83.05	73.24	72.62	72.04	71.09	80.83	80.43	79.76
Wisconsin	57.62	70.63	60.16	60.53	59.74	59.06	72.37	71.82	71.34
Wyoming	50.00	61.59	50.00	50.00	50.00	50.00	65.00	65.00	65.00
American Samoa	50.00	50.00	55.00	55.00	55.00	55.00	68.50	68.50	68.50
Guam	50.00	50.00	55.00	55.00	55.00	55.00	68.50	68.50	68.50
N. Mariana Islands	50.00	50.00	55.00	55.00	55.00	55.00	68.50	68.50	68.50
Puerto Rico	50.00	50.00	55.00	55.00	55.00	55.00	68.50	68.50	68.50
Virgin Islands	50.00	50.00	55.00	55.00	55.00	55.00	68.50	68.50	68.50

Notes: The federal government's share of most Medicaid service costs is determined by the federal medical assistance percentage (FMAP), with some exceptions. For Medicaid administrative costs, the federal share does not vary by state and is generally 50 percent. The enhanced FMAP determines the federal share of both service and administrative costs for CHIP, subject to the availability of funds from a state's federal allotments for CHIP.

FMAPs for Medicaid are generally calculated based on a formula that compares each state's per capita income relative to U.S. per capita income and provides a higher federal match for states with lower per capita incomes, subject to a statutory minimum (50 percent) and maximum (83 percent). The formula for a given state is: FMAP = 1 − ((State per capita income squared / U.S. per capita income squared) x 0.45)

Medicaid exceptions to this formula include the District of Columbia (set in statute at 70 percent) and the territories (set in statute at 55 percent). Other Medicaid exceptions apply to certain services, providers, or situations (e.g., services provided through an Indian Health Service facility receive an FMAP of 100 percent). Enhanced FMAPs for CHIP are calculated by reducing the state share under regular FMAPs for Medicaid by 30 percent.

[1] From the first quarter of FY 2009 through the third quarter of FY 2011, subject to certain requirements, states received a temporary FMAP increase (PL. 111-5 and PL. 111-226). Under the formula used to calculate the temporary increase, states reached their highest FMAPs by the first quarter of FY 2011 (shown here). The temporary increase then phased down in the second and third quarters of FY 2011. FMAPs returned to their regular formula levels in the fourth quarter of FY 2011. The temporary increase did not apply to CHIP.

[2] For certain newly eligible individuals under the Medicaid expansion beginning in 2014, there is an increased FMAP (100 percent in 2014 through 2016, phasing down to 90 percent in 2020 and subsequent years). An increased FMAP is also available for certain states that previously expanded eligibility. (See §§1905(y) and (z) of the Social Security Act.)

[3] Louisiana receives a disaster-recovery state FMAP adjustment for the fourth quarter of FY 2011 and FY 2012-FY 2014 (§1905(aa) of the Social Security Act). PL. 112-96 and PL. 112-141 revised the disaster relief formula, effective October 1, 2012. As a result, HHS has revised the FY 2013 disaster-recovery FMAP adjustment for Louisiana that was published in the *Federal Register* on November 30, 2011.

[4] Texas received a Hurricane Katrina-related FMAP adjustment for FY 2008 (§6053(b) of PL. 109-171).

Source: *Federal Register* notices from the U.S. Department of Health and Human Services

MACStats

TABLE 15. Medicaid as a Share of States' Total Budgets and State-Funded Budgets, State FY 2011

	Total Budget (Including State and Federal Funds)				State-Funded Budget			
	Dollars (millions)	Medicaid	Total spending as a share of total budget[2]		Dollars (millions)	Medicaid	State-funded spending as a share of state-funded budget[2]	
			Elementary and secondary education	Higher education			Elementary and secondary education	Higher education
State								
All states	**$1,662,545**	**23.7%**	**20.2%**	**10.3%**	**$1,096,610**	**13.4%**	**24.1%**	**13.8%**
Alabama	21,021	24.9	24.9	22.5	12,212	11.4	32.0	27.8
Alaska	13,923	9.3	11.0	8.3	10,750	3.7	11.9	9.5
Arizona	28,121	33.9	20.0	13.9	15,762	14.9	27.2	19.9
Arkansas	20,484	21.1	17.2	15.8	13,524	6.6	20.2	23.5
California	215,745	24.2	19.8	7.7	130,981	16.3	26.6	8.2
Colorado	30,917	17.8	23.9	13.6	22,024	12.3	29.5	16.9
Connecticut	25,944	21.6	14.2	10.2	23,370	23.9	13.3	10.3
Delaware	8,412	16.2	24.5	4.7	6,563	7.9	27.7	4.8
District of Columbia[1]	–	–	–	–	–	–	–	–
Florida	65,462	29.2	21.8	8.2	36,111	18.7	28.6	13.5
Georgia	40,458	20.5	25.2	17.1	27,180	8.2	28.2	25.2
Hawaii	11,221	15.9	15.3	9.1	8,667	7.0	16.0	11.3
Idaho	6,602	28.5	25.5	7.6	3,933	15.4	35.4	12.6
Illinois	49,099	32.9	18.9	5.6	36,830	19.4	18.9	6.7
Indiana	26,392	25.0	32.2	7.1	16,440	10.5	45.0	11.2
Iowa	18,051	19.4	17.7	24.6	11,904	10.7	22.3	32.8
Kansas	14,685	18.2	26.0	16.5	10,213	8.8	30.7	19.8
Kentucky	25,433	22.8	19.7	23.8	15,670	8.1	25.1	33.3
Louisiana	31,200	22.1	16.6	7.5	20,231	8.2	19.3	10.8
Maine	8,274	28.3	13.7	3.3	5,274	12.2	20.4	5.0
Maryland	33,851	22.2	21.0	14.5	23,900	12.8	22.7	19.1
Massachusetts	53,302	19.2	11.6	9.9	40,214	10.3	12.3	12.9
Michigan	48,580	24.9	27.6	4.4	28,661	12.1	37.9	7.1
Minnesota	31,401	25.3	22.9	10.2	22,201	14.1	27.6	14.2
Mississippi	22,226	18.5	14.8	13.0	10,530	10.0	23.0	25.6
Missouri	23,103	33.1	23.1	5.1	15,298	23.7	25.3	7.3
Montana	6,164	15.7	15.1	9.8	3,784	5.9	18.0	13.6
Nebraska	9,807	16.4	16.3	22.8	6,585	8.0	16.8	28.2

TABLE 15, Continued

	Total Budget (Including State and Federal Funds)				State-Funded Budget			
	Dollars (millions)	Medicaid	Total spending as a share of total budget[2]		Dollars (millions)	Medicaid	State-funded spending as a share of state-funded budget[2]	
State			Elementary and secondary education	Higher education			Elementary and secondary education	Higher education
Nevada	$8,506	18.3%	21.5%	10.0%	$5,864	10.0%	23.7%	14.5%
New Hampshire	5,340	25.7	22.3	4.0	3,411	17.1	29.1	6.2
New Jersey	47,142	23.3	24.4	8.1	35,098	13.1	28.9	10.8
New Mexico	15,431	22.9	18.9	17.8	9,310	8.5	25.0	23.0
New York	132,765	29.1	20.7	7.1	88,058	12.9	24.3	10.2
North Carolina	51,126	22.1	18.3	12.5	33,518	10.9	23.3	19.0
North Dakota	5,018	14.3	15.8	20.6	3,204	7.0	20.0	27.3
Ohio	60,300	23.2	17.7	4.6	45,868	24.8	18.3	6.0
Oklahoma	21,337	21.2	14.6	16.2	12,101	11.6	18.4	24.0
Oregon	33,442	13.3	11.0	7.2	24,814	5.8	11.6	8.8
Pennsylvania	69,130	31.8	19.5	3.2	39,620	19.7	24.6	5.4
Rhode Island	7,842	25.9	14.4	12.4	5,094	15.9	17.1	18.8
South Carolina	22,188	20.7	17.3	21.0	12,367	10.4	21.2	30.4
South Dakota	3,870	20.7	16.3	18.4	2,191	10.6	17.8	26.8
Tennessee	30,097	29.8	17.3	13.3	16,519	15.6	22.1	22.7
Texas	95,461	24.6	30.0	11.8	59,560	13.5	35.8	18.4
Utah	12,688	14.7	23.2	10.8	9,109	5.7	25.9	14.5
Vermont	4,860	25.5	31.9	2.0	2,894	14.4	47.3	3.4
Virginia	42,332	16.9	15.8	15.3	32,638	9.1	16.6	16.3
Washington	33,621	23.5	23.3	14.2	24,632	16.1	27.0	18.8
West Virginia	21,198	12.9	10.4	12.8	16,738	3.3	10.9	14.2
Wisconsin	42,844	17.0	17.3	13.7	30,608	7.4	21.2	13.2
Wyoming	6,129	9.0	3.8	5.4	4,582	4.7	3.0	6.6

Notes: Total budget includes federal and all other funds. State-funded budget includes state general funds, other state funds, and bonds. Medicaid, elementary and secondary education, and higher education represent the largest total budget shares among functions broken out separately by the National Association of State Budget Officers (NASBO). Functions not shown here are transportation, corrections, public assistance, and all other. Medicaid spending amounts exclude administrative costs but include Medicare Part D "clawback" payments; they also reflect a temporary increase in federal matching funds for Medicaid (see MACStats Table 14 for information).

[1] NASBO does not collect information for the District of Columbia.

[2] Total and state-funded budget shares should be viewed with caution because they reflect varying state practices. For example, Connecticut reports all of its Medicaid spending as state-funded spending due to the direct deposit of federal funds into the State Treasury. In addition, some functions—particularly elementary and secondary education—may also be funded outside of the state budget by local governments.

Source: National Association of State Budget Officers (NASBO), *State expenditure report: Examining fiscal 2010–2012 state spending*, December 2012, http://www.nasbo.org/sites/default/files/State%20Expenditure%20Report_1.pdf

MACStats

TABLE 16. National Health Expenditures by Type and Payer, 2011

	Dollars (billions)						
Type of Expenditure	Total	Medicaid	CHIP	Medicare	Private insurance	Other health insurance[1]	Other third party payers[2]	Out of pocket
National health expenditures	**$2,700.7**	**$407.7**	**$12.0**	**$554.3**	**$896.3**	**$89.8**	**$433.0**	**$307.7**
Hospital	850.6	151.0	3.3	231.3	306.9	50.0	80.0	28.1
Physician and clinical	541.4	44.8	3.0	124.0	249.1	19.5	48.8	52.3
Dental	108.4	7.3	1.1	0.3	52.7	1.4	0.5	45.1
Other professional	73.2	4.9	0.2	15.9	26.7	–	6.5	19.0
Home health	74.3	27.6	0.0	32.9	5.1	0.9	2.2	5.6
Other non-durable medical products	47.0	–	–	–	3.2	–	0.0	43.8
Prescription drugs	263.0	19.0	1.6	63.7	122.2	7.8	3.7	45.0
Durable medical equipment	38.9	4.6	0.1	7.7	4.6	–	0.6	21.3
Nursing care facilities and continuing care retirement communities	149.3	46.1	0.0	37.6	12.4	4.3	9.0	39.9
Other health, residential, and personal care	133.1	69.3	0.9	5.1	6.4	2.9	41.1	7.5
Administration	188.9	33.1	1.8	32.7	110.3	3.0	8.0	–
Public health activity	79.0	–	–	–	–	–	79.0	–
Investment	153.5	–	–	–	–	–	153.5	–

TABLE 16, Continued

Type of Expenditure	Total	Medicaid	CHIP	Medicare	Private insurance	Other health insurance[1]	Other third party payers[2]	Out of pocket
National health expenditures	**100%**	**15.1%**	**0.4%**	**20.5%**	**33.2%**	**3.3%**	**16.0%**	**11.4%**
Hospital	100	17.8	0.4	27.2	36.1	5.9	9.4	3.3
Physician and clinical	100	8.3	0.6	22.9	46.0	3.6	9.0	9.7
Dental	100	6.7	1.1	0.3	48.6	1.3	0.5	41.6
Other professional	100	6.6	0.3	21.7	36.5	–	8.9	26.0
Home health	100	37.1	0.0	44.2	6.9	1.2	3.0	7.6
Other non-durable medical products	100	–	–	6.9	–	–	0.0	93.1
Prescription drugs	100	7.2	0.6	24.2	46.5	3.0	1.4	17.1
Durable medical equipment	100	11.9	0.3	19.7	11.7	–	1.5	54.9
Nursing care facilities and continuing care retirement communities	100	30.9	0.0	25.2	8.3	2.9	6.1	26.7
Other health, residential, and personal care	100	52.0	0.7	3.8	4.8	2.2	30.9	5.6
Administration	100	17.5	1.0	17.3	58.4	1.6	4.2	–
Public health activity	100	–	–	–	–	–	100.0	–
Investment	100	–	–	–	–	–	100.0	–

Notes: Figures for nursing care facilities and continuing retirement communities and other health, residential, and personal care reflect new data and methods as of 2011. In prior releases, Medicaid accounted for about 40 percent of nursing home expenditures and about three-quarters of other personal health care expenditures. Other professional includes services provided in establishments operated by health practitioners other than physicians and dentists, including those provided by private-duty nurses, chiropractors, podiatrists, optometrists, and physical, occupational, and speech therapists, among others. Other non-durable medical products includes the retail sales of non-prescription drugs and medical sundries. Durable medical equipment includes retail sales of items such as contact lenses, eyeglasses, and other ophthalmic products, surgical and orthopedic products, hearing aids, wheelchairs, and medical equipment rentals. Nursing care facilities and continuing care retirement communities includes nursing and rehabilitative services provided in freestanding nursing home facilities that are generally provided for an extended period of time by registered or licensed practical nurses and other staff. Other health, residential, and personal care includes spending for Medicaid home and community-based waivers, care provided in residential facilities for people with intellectual disabilities or mental health and substance abuse disorders, ambulance services, school health, and worksite health care. Administration category includes the administrative cost of health care programs (e.g., Medicare and Medicaid) and the net cost of private health insurance (administrative costs, as well as additions to reserves, rate credits and dividends, premium taxes, and plan profits or losses). Zeroes indicate amounts less than $0.05 billion or 0.05 percent that round to zero. Dashes indicate amounts that are true zeroes.

1 U.S. Department of Defense and U.S. Department of Veterans' Affairs.

2 Includes all other public and private programs and expenditures except for out-of-pocket amounts.

Sources: Office of the Actuary (OACT), Centers for Medicare & Medicaid Services, *National health expenditures by type of service and source of funds: Calendar years 1960-2011*, January 2013, http://www.cms.gov/Research-Statistics-Data-and-Systems/Statistics-Trends-and-Reports/NationalHealthExpendData/Downloads/NHE2011.zip and OACT, *National health expenditure accounts: Methodology paper, 2011*, 2013, http://www.cms.gov/Research-Statistics-Data-and-Systems/Statistics-Trends-and-Reports/NationalHealthExpendData/Downloads/dsm-11.pdf

MACStats

TABLE 17. Historical and Projected National Health Expenditures by Payer for Selected Years, 1970–2021

	Dollars (billions)					
	Total	Medicaid and CHIP	Medicare	Private insurance	Other health insurance[1]	Other third party payers[2]	Out of pocket

	Total	Medicaid and CHIP	Medicare	Private insurance	Other health insurance[1]	Other third party payers[2]	Out of pocket
Historical							
1970	$75	$5	$8	$15	$3	$18	$25
1975	134	13	16	30	6	30	37
1980	256	26	37	69	10	55	58
1985	445	41	72	131	15	89	96
1990	724	74	110	234	21	146	139
1995	1,027	145	184	327	27	198	146
2000	1,377	203	225	459	33	255	202
2001	1,493	228	248	502	37	269	209
2002	1,638	254	265	561	42	294	222
2003	1,775	275	283	616	49	316	236
2004	1,902	298	311	660	53	330	248
2005	2,030	317	340	704	57	350	263
2006	2,163	315	404	742	62	370	272
2007	2,298	335	434	779	66	398	286
2008	2,407	355	468	809	72	408	293
2009	2,501	387	500	835	79	407	293
2010	2,600	409	522	864	84	421	299
2011	2,701	420	554	896	90	433	308
Projected							
2012	2,809	472	591	889	94	451	312
2013	2,915	505	598	925	99	465	323
2014	3,130	595	635	998	104	481	318
2015	3,308	637	666	1,060	110	504	329
2016	3,514	688	707	1,130	117	532	340
2017	3,723	729	755	1,191	125	565	359
2018	3,952	777	809	1,253	134	599	382
2019	4,207	832	868	1,329	143	632	403
2020	4,487	895	935	1,412	153	667	426
2021	4,781	963	1,007	1,495	163	703	449

TABLE 17, Continued

	Total	Medicaid and CHIP	Medicare	Share of Total Private insurance	Other health insurance[1]	Other third party payers[2]	Out of pocket
Historical							
1970	100%	7.1%	10.2%	20.6%	4.4%	24.2%	33.4%
1975	100	10.1	12.2	22.8	4.5	22.5	28.0
1980	100	10.2	14.6	27.0	3.8	21.6	22.8
1985	100	9.2	16.2	29.5	3.4	20.1	21.6
1990	100	10.2	15.2	32.3	3.0	20.2	19.1
1995	100	14.1	17.9	31.8	2.6	19.3	14.2
2000	100	14.8	16.3	33.3	2.4	18.5	14.6
2001	100	15.3	16.6	33.6	2.4	18.0	14.0
2002	100	15.5	16.2	34.3	2.6	17.9	13.5
2003	100	15.5	15.9	34.7	2.8	17.8	13.3
2004	100	15.7	16.4	34.7	2.8	17.4	13.1
2005	100	15.6	16.7	34.7	2.8	17.2	12.9
2006	100	14.6	18.7	34.3	2.8	17.1	12.6
2007	100	14.6	18.9	33.9	2.9	17.3	12.4
2008	100	14.8	19.5	33.6	3.0	17.0	12.2
2009	100	15.5	20.0	33.4	3.2	16.3	11.7
2010	100	15.7	20.1	33.2	3.2	16.2	11.5
2011	100	15.5	20.5	33.2	3.3	16.0	11.4
Projected							
2012	100	16.8	21.0	31.6	3.4	16.0	11.1
2013	100	17.3	20.5	31.7	3.4	16.0	11.1
2014	100	19.0	20.3	31.9	3.3	15.4	10.2
2015	100	19.3	20.1	32.1	3.3	15.2	9.9
2016	100	19.6	20.1	32.2	3.3	15.1	9.7
2017	100	19.6	20.3	32.0	3.4	15.2	9.7
2018	100	19.6	20.5	31.7	3.4	15.2	9.7
2019	100	19.8	20.6	31.6	3.4	15.0	9.6
2020	100	19.9	20.8	31.5	3.4	14.9	9.5
2021	100	20.2	21.1	31.3	3.4	14.7	9.4

Note: Historical data were released in 2013; projections data were released in 2012 and may therefore reflect different assumptions than those used to produce the current historical data.

1 U.S. Department of Defense and U.S. Department of Veterans' Affairs.

2 Includes all other public and private programs and expenditures except for out-of-pocket amounts.

Sources: Office of the Actuary (OACT), Centers for Medicare & Medicaid Services, *National health expenditures by type of service and source of funds: Calendar years 1960–2011*, January 2013, http://www.cms.gov/Research-Statistics-Data-and-Systems/Statistics-Trends-and-Reports/NationalHealthExpendData/Downloads/NHE2011.zip, for historical; OACT, *National health expenditure (NHE) amounts by type of expenditure and source of funds: Calendar years 1970–2021* in projections format, July 2012 and MACPAC communication with OACT, December 2012, for projected

MACStats

TABLE 18. Characteristics of Non-Institutionalized Individuals by Source of Health Insurance, 2012

	Total all ages	All Ages				Total age 0-18	Age 0-18			
		Private	Medicaid/CHIP	Medicare	Uninsured		Private	Medicaid/CHIP	Medicare	Uninsured
Within Age Group[1]										
Number of People (millions)	307.9	185.7	50.5	45.9	45.0	78.0	41.9	28.9	0.3	5.5
Share of Population	100.0%	60.3%*	16.4%	14.9%*	14.6%*	100.0%	53.7%*	37.0%	0.4%*	7.0%*
Within Insurance Coverage Type										
Gender (%)										
Male	48.9*	49.0*	44.3	44.4	53.7*	51.2	51.7	50.4	48.9	50.5
Female	51.1*	51.0*	55.7	55.6	46.3*	48.8	48.3	49.6	51.1	49.5
Family Income (%)[2]										
<100% of poverty	14.7*	4.0*	46.7	11.1*	27.4*	20.8*	3.7*	47.7	41.6	24.5*
100 – 199% of poverty	19.2*	11.2*	33.2	24.2*	33.6	22.5*	12.8*	35.7	35.3	34.2
200+ % of poverty	66.0*	84.8*	20.1	64.7*	39.0*	56.7*	83.5*	16.7	23.0	41.4*
Race/Ethnicity (%)										
Hispanic	16.9*	10.3*	29.3	7.6*	33.5*	23.6*	13.3*	34.8	41.5	41.0
White, non-Hispanic	63.6*	73.4*	40.6	77.6*	46.1*	53.8*	69.0*	35.7	25.6	39.0
Black, non-Hispanic	11.9*	8.6*	21.7	9.9*	13.3*	13.4*	8.0*	21.7	30.8	9.8*
Other races and multiple races	7.6	7.7	8.4	4.8*	7.1	9.1	9.8*	7.8	†	10.2
Health Status (%)										
Excellent or very good	65.6*	72.1*	58.5	39.5*	59.0	82.3*	88.1*	73.0	81.4	83.4*
Good	24.3*	21.8*	26.1	33.3*	28.5*	15.6*	10.9*	23.1	14.5	14.3*
Fair or poor	10.1*	6.1*	15.4	27.2*	12.5*	2.1*	0.9*	3.9	†	2.3*
Place of Residence (%)[3]										
Large MSA	54.4	56.0	52.2	47.9	52.9	54.8	58.0*	51.4	59.1	51.9
Small MSA	29.8	29.7	29.5	31.1	28.7	29.9	29.0	30.0	35.5	30.8
Not in MSA	15.8	14.3*	18.3	21.0	18.4	15.3*	12.9*	18.6	†	17.3

TABLE 18, Continued

	Total age 19-64	Age 19-64				Total age 65 and over	Age 65 and Over			
		Private	Medicaid/CHIP	Medicare	Uninsured		Private	Medicaid/CHIP	Medicare	Uninsured
Within Age Group[1]										
Number of People (millions)	188.5	122.3	18.5	6.2	39.2	41.4	21.4	3.1	39.0	0.4
Share of Population	100.0%	64.9%*	9.8%	3.3%*	20.8%*	100.0%	51.7%*	7.6%	94.3%*	0.9%*
Within Insurance Coverage Type										
Gender (%)										
Male	48.9*	49.0*	36.5	48.4*	54.1*	44.0*	44.3*	33.8	43.7*	56.9*
Female	51.1*	51.0*	63.5	51.6*	45.9*	56.0*	55.7*	66.2	56.3*	43.1*
Family Income (%)[2]										
<100% of poverty	13.7*	4.2*	47.0	31.3*	27.8*	7.8*	2.9*	35.7	7.5*	24.6
100 – 199% of poverty	17.2*	9.7*	29.5	32.7	33.5*	22.5*	17.2*	32.7	22.7*	36.7
200+% of poverty	69.1*	86.1*	23.5	36.0*	38.7*	69.7*	79.8*	31.6	69.8*	38.7
Race/Ethnicity (%)										
Hispanic	16.3*	10.5*	21.5	10.7*	32.4*	7.3*	3.3*	24.2	6.9*	34.0
White, non-Hispanic	64.2*	72.6*	46.6	64.4*	47.1	79.2*	86.4*	50.4	80.2*	47.2
Black, non-Hispanic	12.0*	9.2*	22.8	19.2	13.8*	8.5*	6.3*	15.5	8.3*	10.9
Other races and multiple races	7.5	7.6	9.0	5.8*	6.6*	5.0*	3.9*	9.9	4.7*	7.9
Health Status (%)										
Excellent or very good	63.5*	70.9*	41.2	13.5*	55.8*	43.6*	47.8*	25.7	43.3*	42.1*
Good	25.7*	23.4*	30.3	26.8	30.5	34.3*	34.3*	29.3	34.5*	28.9
Fair or poor	10.7*	5.7*	28.5	59.7*	13.8*	22.2*	17.9*	44.9	22.2*	29.0*
Place of Residence (%)[3]										
Large MSA	54.4	57.1	53.5	46.6*	53.0	48.8	46.0	52.2	48.0	62.0
Small MSA	29.6	29.5	29.7	29.7	28.5	30.7	32.2*	24.5	31.3	16.1
Not in MSA	14.9	13.4*	16.8	23.7*	18.5	20.4	21.8	23.3	20.7	21.9

TABLE 18, Continued

Notes:

1 Sum of health insurance coverage types may not add to total for each age group because individuals may have multiple sources of coverage and because not all types of coverage (e.g., military) are displayed. Insurance coverage is measured at the time of the interview. Private health insurance coverage excludes plans that paid for only one type of service, such as accidents or dental care. Medicaid/CHIP also includes persons covered by other public programs, excluding Medicare (e.g., other state-sponsored health plans); nevertheless, as discussed in Table 1, survey data tend to report lower Medicaid/CHIP enrollment than administrative data. Individuals were defined as uninsured if they did not have any private health insurance, Medicare, Medicaid/CHIP, state-sponsored or other government-sponsored health plans, or a military plan. Individuals were also defined as uninsured if they had only Indian Health Service coverage or had only a private plan that paid for one type of service, such as accidents or dental care.

2 For numerous reasons, poverty status shown here may differ from levels calculated by state Medicaid and CHIP programs. While these survey results show coverage as of the time of the survey in 2012, family income is for the prior year, 2011. In 2011, 100 percent of poverty using the U.S. Census Bureau's poverty threshold was $17,916 for a family of three. The poverty threshold differs from the federal poverty guidelines used for Medicaid and CHIP eligibility determinations. (The family income results shown here exclude the 11 percent of respondents with unknown poverty status.) In addition, data from surveys like the National Health Interview Survey tend to include more income and more relatives as part of the family unit, compared to how income is counted for Medicaid and CHIP.

3 MSA is a metropolitan statistical area with a population size of 50,000 or more persons. Large MSAs have a population size of 1,000,000 or more; small MSAs have a population size between 50,000 and 1,000,000.

† Sample size is not sufficient to support published estimates.

* Difference from Medicaid/CHIP is statistically significant at the 95 percent confidence level.

Source: Analysis of National Health Interview Survey (NHIS) data by the National Center for Health Statistics (NCHS) for MACPAC, January 2013; the estimates for 2012 are based on data collected from January through June, based on household interviews of a sample of the civilian non-institutionalized population

MAC Stats

MAC Stats

TABLE 19. Income as a Percentage of the Federal Poverty Level (FPL) for Various Family Sizes, 2013

States		Annual					States		Monthly				
		Family size				Amount for each additional family member			Family size				Amount for each additional family member
		1	2	3	4				1	2	3	4	
Lower 48 states and DC	100% FPL	$11,490	$15,510	$19,530	$23,550	$4,020	Lower 48 states and DC	100% FPL	$958	$1,293	$1,628	$1,963	$335
	133% FPL	15,282	20,628	25,975	31,322	5,347		133% FPL	1,273	1,719	2,165	2,610	446
	138% FPL	15,856	21,404	26,951	32,499	5,548		138% FPL	1,321	1,784	2,246	2,708	462
	150% FPL	17,235	23,265	29,295	35,325	6,030		150% FPL	1,436	1,939	2,441	2,944	503
	185% FPL	21,257	28,694	36,131	43,568	7,437		185% FPL	1,771	2,391	3,011	3,631	620
	200% FPL	22,980	31,020	39,060	47,100	8,040		200% FPL	1,915	2,585	3,255	3,925	670
	250% FPL	28,725	38,775	48,825	58,875	10,050		250% FPL	2,394	3,231	4,069	4,906	838
	300% FPL	34,470	46,530	58,590	70,650	12,060		300% FPL	2,873	3,878	4,883	5,888	1,005
	400% FPL	45,960	62,040	78,120	94,200	16,080		400% FPL	3,830	5,170	6,510	7,850	1,340
Alaska	100% FPL	$14,350	$19,380	$24,410	$29,440	$5,030	Alaska	100% FPL	$1,196	$1,615	$2,034	$2,453	$419
	133% FPL	19,086	25,775	32,465	39,155	6,690		133% FPL	1,590	2,148	2,705	3,263	557
	138% FPL	19,803	26,744	33,686	40,627	6,941		138% FPL	1,650	2,229	2,807	3,386	578
	150% FPL	21,525	29,070	36,615	44,160	7,545		150% FPL	1,794	2,423	3,051	3,680	629
	185% FPL	26,548	35,853	45,159	54,464	9,306		185% FPL	2,212	2,988	3,763	4,539	775
	200% FPL	28,700	38,760	48,820	58,880	10,060		200% FPL	2,392	3,230	4,068	4,907	838
	250% FPL	35,875	48,450	61,025	73,600	12,575		250% FPL	2,990	4,038	5,085	6,133	1,048
	300% FPL	43,050	58,140	73,230	88,320	15,090		300% FPL	3,588	4,845	6,103	7,360	1,258
	400% FPL	57,400	77,520	97,640	117,760	20,120		400% FPL	4,783	6,460	8,137	9,813	1,677
Hawaii	100% FPL	$13,230	$17,850	$22,470	$27,090	$4,620	Hawaii	100% FPL	$1,103	$1,488	$1,873	$2,258	$385
	133% FPL	17,596	23,741	29,885	36,030	6,145		133% FPL	1,466	1,978	2,490	3,002	512
	138% FPL	18,257	24,633	31,009	37,384	6,376		138% FPL	1,521	2,053	2,584	3,115	531
	150% FPL	19,845	26,775	33,705	40,635	6,930		150% FPL	1,654	2,231	2,809	3,386	578
	185% FPL	24,476	33,023	41,570	50,117	8,547		185% FPL	2,040	2,752	3,464	4,176	712
	200% FPL	26,460	35,700	44,940	54,180	9,240		200% FPL	2,205	2,975	3,745	4,515	770
	250% FPL	33,075	44,625	56,175	67,725	11,550		250% FPL	2,756	3,719	4,681	5,644	963
	300% FPL	39,690	53,550	67,410	81,270	13,860		300% FPL	3,308	4,463	5,618	6,773	1,155
	400% FPL	52,920	71,400	89,880	108,360	18,480		400% FPL	4,410	5,950	7,490	9,030	1,540

Notes: The FPLs shown here are based on the U.S. Department of Health and Human Services 2013 federal poverty guidelines. These differ slightly from the U.S. Census Bureau's federal poverty thresholds, which are used mainly for statistical purposes. The separate poverty guidelines for Alaska and Hawaii reflect Office of Economic Opportunity administrative practice beginning in the 1966–1970 period.

Source: U.S. Department of Health and Human Services (HHS), Annual update of the HHS poverty guidelines. *Federal Register* 78 (January 24): 5183, 2013

MACStats

TABLE 20. Supplemental Payments by State and Category, FY 2012 (millions)

State[1]	Inpatient and Outpatient Hospital[2]				Mental Health Facilities[3]		
	DSH payments	Non-DSH supplemental payments	Total Medicaid payments	Supplemental payments as % of total	DSH payments	Total Medicaid payments	Supplemental payments as % of total
All states	$14,345.0	$18,339.6	$85,479.0	38.2%	$2,731.1	$6,120.4	44.6%
Alabama	455.2	359.2	1,896.0	43.0	3.3	68.9	4.8
Alaska	6.1	–	295.7	2.1	13.8	31.1	44.3
Arizona	168.1	245.8	895.6	46.2	26.5	28.4	93.6
Arkansas	60.6	316.2	978.1	38.5	0.8	155.8	0.5
California	2,101.2	2,397.8	11,449.0	39.3	0.3	387.4	0.1
Colorado	189.5	783.8	1,598.6	60.9	–	3.8	–
Connecticut	372.5	163.8	1,738.6	30.8	105.6	178.7	59.1
Delaware	7.0	0.0	64.5	10.9	5.6	6.4	88.6
District of Columbia	54.6	9.2	411.6	15.5	6.5	18.3	35.8
Florida	245.6	937.0	4,936.4	24.0	119.8	188.6	63.5
Georgia	415.8	79.4	2,130.3	23.2	–	37.3	–
Hawaii	–	27.3	75.2	36.3	–	–	–
Idaho	23.4	28.6	386.9	13.4	–	1.7	–
Illinois	355.2	1,607.3	4,875.3	40.3	88.8	160.5	55.3
Indiana[6]	–	174.1	1,589.9	11.0	-1.3	32.0	-4.0
Iowa	52.0	27.0	810.4	9.7	–	20.8	–
Kansas	49.7	58.5	415.3	26.0	24.5	70.7	34.6
Kentucky	171.2	25.2	615.9	31.9	37.3	66.7	55.9
Louisiana	657.3	370.5	2,114.7	48.6	75.7	90.4	83.8
Maine	–	4.0	481.9	0.8	41.2	88.5	46.6
Maryland	25.7	46.0	996.9	7.2	10.6	118.2	9.0
Massachusetts	–	649.5	2,204.3	29.5	–	113.1	–
Michigan	175.0	707.1	1,628.0	54.2	101.0	155.6	64.9
Minnesota	47.4	54.2	634.8	16.0	0.2	93.4	0.2
Mississippi	210.5	397.4	1,627.8	37.3	–	69.4	–
Missouri	532.8	117.4	3,017.0	21.5	222.8	258.5	86.2
Montana	17.1	1.9	252.7	7.5	–	15.7	–
Nebraska[7]	38.7	-1.1	277.5	13.5	3.3	17.5	18.7
Nevada	85.5	137.8	498.0	44.9	–	41.6	–

TABLE 20, Continued

	Inpatient and Outpatient Hospital[2]				Mental Health Facilities[3]		
State[1]	DSH payments	Non-DSH supplemental payments	Total Medicaid payments	Supplemental payments as % of total	DSH payments	Total Medicaid payments	Supplemental payments as % of total
New Hampshire	$22.2	–	$179.6	12.4%	$19.8	$27.3	72.4%
New Jersey	885.4	$255.7	1,742.9	65.5	357.4	462.7	77.2
New Mexico	56.4	348.8	512.7	79.0	–	4.2	–
New York	2,684.7	437.7	10,145.5	30.8	565.7	1,080.1	52.4
North Carolina	310.1	2,062.9	4,413.4	53.8	0.2	99.8	0.2
North Dakota	0.2	2.9	123.1	2.5	1.0	10.0	9.9
Ohio	544.5	325.1	2,209.7	39.4	–	489.7	–
Oklahoma	35.3	503.7	1,581.0	34.1	0.8	69.9	1.2
Oregon	49.3	92.7	366.1	38.8	20.0	21.3	93.6
Pennsylvania	779.9	357.6	2,071.5	54.9	381.8	451.4	84.6
Rhode Island	127.7	12.0	342.3	40.8	–	5.5	–
South Carolina	404.8	59.7	1,121.0	41.4	52.3	92.7	56.5
South Dakota	–	–	184.7	–	0.8	3.4	22.3
Tennessee	102.3	1,154.1	1,351.0	93.0	–	31.9	–
Texas	1,223.5	2,353.8	5,939.1	60.2	292.5	318.1	92.0
Utah	31.0	230.4	598.3	43.7	1.9	16.9	11.0
Vermont	37.4	0.0	43.5	86.1	–	0.0	–
Virginia	207.9	233.8	1,054.6	41.9	6.7	142.5	4.7
Washington	267.6	–	1,346.6	19.9	124.9	148.7	84.0
West Virginia	56.6	130.7	480.0	39.0	18.9	101.6	18.6
Wisconsin	0.1	39.4	658.3	6.0	–	15.2	–
Wyoming	0.5	13.7	116.8	12.1	–	8.7	–

MACStats

TABLE 20, Continued. Supplemental Payments by State and Category, FY 2012 (millions)

State[1]	Nursing Facilities and ICF-ID[4]			Physician and Other Practitioner[5]		
	Non-DSH supplemental payments	Total Medicaid payments	Supplemental payments as % of total	Non-DSH supplemental payments	Total Medicaid payments	Supplemental payments as % of total
All states	$2,377.2	$64,039.5	3.7%	$891.4	$13,499.7	6.6%
Alabama	—	930.6	—	—	352.4	—
Alaska	—	131.7	—	—	123.3	—
Arizona	—	35.3	—	—	34.1	—
Arkansas	—	832.9	—	31.1	300.4	10.4
California	475.9	5,412.2	8.8	—	901.7	—
Colorado	95.5	663.5	14.4	5.2	295.3	1.8
Connecticut	—	1,529.8	—	—	298.5	—
Delaware	—	142.2	—	—	18.0	—
District of Columbia	—	285.9	—	—	47.2	—
Florida	7.8	3,125.0	0.3	68.2	1,120.2	6.1
Georgia	283.2	1,301.5	21.8	59.9	409.9	14.6
Hawaii	0.6	10.1	6.1	—	2.9	—
Idaho	45.4	243.4	18.6	—	100.6	—
Illinois	—	2,441.4	—	—	755.6	—
Indiana	268.1	1,745.2	15.4	85.4	233.1	36.6
Iowa	—	877.2	—	—	246.7	—
Kansas	8.5	505.4	1.7	16.7	101.8	16.4
Kentucky	0.6	1,004.6	0.1	—	116.2	—
Louisiana	—	1,330.9	—	48.6	411.3	11.8
Maine	—	303.7	—	0.0	134.5	0.0
Maryland	5.7	1,153.2	0.5	—	93.0	—
Massachusetts	0.1	1,800.0	0.0	29.1	310.4	9.4
Michigan	342.8	1,740.8	19.7	201.3	356.9	56.4
Minnesota	—	940.5	—	1.4	362.3	0.4
Mississippi	17.8	1,027.1	1.7	—	293.5	—
Missouri	—	1,297.5	—	—	34.5	—
Montana	—	171.8	—	—	62.4	—
Nebraska	—	381.8	—	—	65.5	—
Nevada	—	210.9	—	2.4	100.3	2.4
New Hampshire	—	327.8	—	—	62.6	—
New Jersey	—	2,412.8	—	—	48.6	—
New Mexico	—	27.5	—	14.6	89.8	16.2
New York	60.2	10,447.1	0.6	—	575.1	—

TABLE 20, Continued

	Nursing Facilities and ICF-ID[4]			Physician and Other Practitioner[5]		
State[1]	Non-DSH supplemental payments	Total Medicaid payments	Supplemental payments as % of total	Non-DSH supplemental payments	Total Medicaid payments	Supplemental payments as % of total
North Carolina	–	$1,668.7	–	$108.6	$1,091.3	10.0%
North Dakota	$2.2	293.5	0.7%	–	54.0	–
Ohio	82.1	3,289.6	2.5	–	318.4	–
Oklahoma	–	611.4	–	–	481.1	–
Oregon	–	330.7	–	–	49.7	–
Pennsylvania	592.4	4,171.7	14.2	–	220.7	–
Rhode Island	–	333.2	–	–	12.7	–
South Carolina	25.7	708.4	3.6	36.0	214.3	16.8
South Dakota	–	164.6	–	–	58.2	–
Tennessee	–	213.4	–	–	26.7	–
Texas	–	3,464.9	–	76.2	1,621.1	4.7
Utah	–	236.5	–	16.0	118.9	13.4
Vermont	0.1	115.9	0.1	–	1.8	–
Virginia	2.7	1,120.9	0.2	25.4	230.2	11.0
Washington	–	726.1	–	38.8	249.9	15.5
West Virginia	–	599.3	–	26.7	155.1	17.2
Wisconsin	39.4	1,085.2	3.6	–	65.3	–
Wyoming	20.4	114.3	17.9	–	71.7	–

Notes: Includes federal and state funds. Excludes payments made under managed care arrangements. All amounts in this table are as reported by states in CMS-64 data during the fiscal year to obtain federal matching funds; they include expenditures for the current fiscal year and adjustments to expenditures for prior fiscal years that may be positive or negative. Amounts reported by states for any given category (e.g., inpatient hospital) sometimes show substantial annual fluctuations. Data limitations: CMS only began to require separate reporting of non-disproportionate share hospital (non-DSH) supplemental payments in FY 2010 and is continuing to work with states to standardize this reporting. As a result, the information presented below may not reflect a consistent classification of supplemental payment spending across states. Reporting is expected to improve over time. Zeroes indicate amounts less than $0.05 million that round to zero. Dashes indicate amounts that are true zeroes.

1 Not all states have certified their CMS-64 Financial Management Report (FMR) submissions as of February 25, 2013. Idaho's 3rd quarter submission is not certified; Alabama and California's 4th quarter submissions are not certified. Figures presented in this table may change once all states have finalized and certified their expenditure data.

2 Includes inpatient, outpatient, critical access hospital, and emergency hospital categories in the CMS-64 data. The CMS-64 instructions to states note that DSH payments are those made in accordance with Section 1923 of the Social Security Act (the Act). Non-DSH supplemental payments are described in the CMS-64 instructions to states as those made in addition to the standard fee schedule or other standard payment for a given service. They include payments made under institutional upper payment limit rules and payments to hospitals for graduate medical education.

3 Includes inpatient psychiatric services for individuals under age 21 and inpatient hospital or nursing facility services for individuals age 65 or older in an institution for mental diseases. The CMS-64 instructions to states note that DSH payments are those made in accordance with Section 1923 of the Act. States are not instructed to break out non-DSH supplemental payments for mental health facilities.

4 Includes nursing facility and intermediate care facility for persons with intellectual disabilities. Non-DSH supplemental payments are described in the CMS-64 instructions to states as payments that are made in addition to the standard fee schedule or other standard payment for a given service, including payments made under institutional upper payment limit rules.

5 Includes the physician and other practitioner categories in CMS-64 data; excludes additional categories (e.g., dental, nurse midwife, nurse practitioner) for which states are not instructed to break out supplemental payments. The CMS-64 instructions to states describe supplemental payments as those that are made in addition to the standard fee schedule payment. Unlike for institutional providers, there is not a regulatory upper payment limit for physicians and other practitioners.

6 Indiana reported negative DSH mental health facility payments, creating a negative percentage.

7 Nebraska reported negative non-DSH supplemental payments for inpatient hospitals.

Source: MACPAC analysis of CMS-64 Financial Management Report (FMR) net expenditure data as of February 2013

TABLE 21. Federal CHIP Allotments, FY 2012 and FY 2013 (millions)

State	FY 2012 CHIP Allotments	FY 2012 Federal CHIP Spending	FY 2013 Allotment Increase Factor	FY 2013 Federal CHIP Allotments	Change in Federal CHIP Allotments Between FY 2012 and FY 2013
A	B	C	D	E = C x D	F = (E/B) - 1
Alabama	$168.1	$156.7	1.0394	$162.8	-3.1%
Alaska	21.0	19.8	1.0394	20.6	-2.1
Arizona	64.6	24.4	1.0394	25.4	-60.7
Arkansas	95.4	99.2	1.0394	103.1	8.1
California	1,314.3	1,246.8	1.0394	1,296.0	-1.4
Colorado	130.4	126.3	1.0442	131.8	1.1
Connecticut	32.7	39.8	1.0394	41.3	26.4
Delaware	14.2	15.1	1.0394	15.7	11.1
District of Columbia	12.6	13.9	1.0708	14.9	17.9
Florida	339.8	345.4	1.0394	359.0	5.7
Georgia	250.9	271.6	1.0411	282.7	12.7
Hawaii	34.8	24.8	1.0412	25.8	-25.8
Idaho	37.9	34.6	1.0394	36.0	-5.2
Illinois	285.1	265.1	1.0394	275.6	-3.4
Indiana	98.7	139.4	1.0394	144.9	46.8
Iowa	115.3	89.0	1.0394	92.5	-19.7
Kansas	58.8	53.3	1.0394	55.4	-5.7
Kentucky	135.5	142.3	1.0394	147.9	9.2
Louisiana	195.2	165.1	1.0409	171.9	-11.9
Maine	37.0	30.3	1.0394	31.5	-15.0
Maryland	176.3	154.4	1.0394	160.5	-9.0
Massachusetts	330.8	318.3	1.0394	330.9	0.0
Michigan	126.2	52.7	1.0394	54.8	-56.6
Minnesota	21.4	30.9	1.0394	32.1	50.0
Mississippi	167.7	170.2	1.0394	176.9	5.5
Missouri	117.6	118.3	1.0394	122.9	4.5
Montana	40.1	57.1	1.0394	59.4	47.9
Nebraska	50.1	40.8	1.0420	42.5	-15.3
Nevada	25.1	30.3	1.0394	31.5	25.2
New Hampshire	13.4	17.5	1.0394	18.2	36.0
New Jersey	618.0	615.9	1.0394	640.2	3.6
New Mexico	258.7	119.1	1.0429	124.2	-52.0
New York	556.8	557.8	1.0394	579.8	4.1
North Carolina	401.2	292.0	1.0418	304.2	-24.2
North Dakota	16.1	16.5	1.0485	17.3	7.8
Ohio	290.1	323.3	1.0394	336.1	15.8

TABLE 21, Continued

State	FY 2012 CHIP Allotments	FY 2012 Federal CHIP Spending	FY 2013 Allotment Increase Factor	FY 2013 Federal CHIP Allotments	Change in Federal CHIP Allotments Between FY 2012 and FY 2013
A	B	C	D	E = C x D	F = (E/B) - 1
Oklahoma	$126.9	$109.2	1.0456	$114.2	-10.0%
Oregon	95.4	138.4	1.0394	143.9	50.9
Pennsylvania	335.9	294.1	1.0394	305.7	-9.0
Rhode Island	31.7	38.0	1.0394	39.5	24.8
South Carolina	102.5	94.4	1.0413	98.3	-4.1
South Dakota	21.1	18.7	1.0422	19.4	-8.0
Tennessee	145.6	192.6	1.0394	200.2	37.5
Texas	882.6	849.1	1.0500	891.5	1.0
Utah	67.8	59.6	1.0483	62.5	-7.9
Vermont	6.9	12.5	1.0394	13.0	88.0
Virginia	184.0	179.4	1.0400	186.6	1.4
Washington	47.6	93.0	1.0426	96.9	103.6
West Virginia	43.1	46.4	1.0394	48.3	12.1
Wisconsin	107.2	99.1	1.0394	103.0	-3.9
Wyoming	10.4	10.4	1.0394	10.8	3.1
Subtotal	**$8,860.5**	**$8,452.7**	**–**	**$8,799.9**	**-0.7%**
American Samoa	1.3	1.3	1.0394	1.3	3.9
Guam	4.4	4.4	1.0394	4.5	3.9
N. Mariana Islands	0.9	0.9	1.0394	0.9	3.9
Puerto Rico	103.9	127.6	1.0394	132.7	27.7
Virgin Islands	–	–	1.0394	–	–
Total	**$8,970.9**	**$8,586.8**	**–**	**$8,939.4**	**-0.4%**

Note: For even-numbered years (e.g., FY 2012), federal CHIP allotments are based on each state's prior-year allotment. For odd-numbered years (e.g., FY 2013), allotments are rebased, based on each state's prior-year spending. Although 2009 legislation provided federal appropriations of $17.4 billion for CHIP allotments in FY 2013, this table shows that only $8.9 billion was necessary for the allotments. While the total allotments for FY 2013 are similar to FY 2012 (0.3 percent difference nationally), the rebasing caused substantial changes for many individual states' allotment levels. Zeroes indicate amounts less than 0.05 percent that round to zero. Dashes indicate amounts that are true zeroes or not applicable.

Sources: MACPAC analysis of Medicaid and CHIP Budget Expenditure System (MBES/CBES) data from the Centers for Medicare & Medicaid Services (CMS) as of February 2013; MACPAC communication with CMS in March 2013

MACStats

TABLE 22. Federal CHIPRA Bonus Payments (millions)

State	FY 2009 CHIPRA bonus payments	FY 2010 CHIPRA bonus payments	FY 2011 CHIPRA bonus payments	Preliminary FY 2012 CHIPRA bonus payments	12 months of continuous eligibility	Liberalization of asset requirements	Elimination of in-person interview	Joint application and renewal form	Automatic administrative renewal	Presumptive eligibility	Express lane	Premium assistance
Total	$37.1	$167.2	$303.5	$306.0	14	22	23	23	18	11	6	5
AL[1]	1.5	5.7	20.4	15.6	✓	✓	✓	✓	✓	—	—	—
AK	0.7	4.9	5.7	4.0	—	✓	✓	✓	✓	✓	—	—
CO	—	18.2	32.9	42.9	—	✓	✓	✓	✓	✓	✓	—
CT	—	—	5.2	2.0	—	✓	✓	✓	—	—	✓	—
GA	—	—	4.9	1.9	✓	✓	✓	✓	✓	—	—	—
ID	—	0.9	0.5	1.5	✓	✓	✓	✓	✓	✓	—	—
IL	9.5	15.3	15.3	12.9	✓	✓	✓	✓	✓	✓	—	—
IA	—	7.7	10.0	11.2	✓	✓	✓	✓	✓	—	—	—
KS	1.2	5.5	6.0	12.3	✓	✓	✓	✓	—	—	—	—
LA	1.5	3.7	1.9	—	—	—	✓	✓	✓	✓	—	—
MD	—	11.4	28.0	36.5	—	✓	✓	✓	✓	✓	—	—
MI	4.7	8.4	6.9	3.3	—	✓	✓	✓	✓	✓	—	—
MT	—	—	5.0	4.8	—	✓	✓	✓	—	✓	—	—
NJ	3.1	8.8	17.6	22.2	✓	✓	✓	✓	✓	✓	—	—
NM	5.4	9.0	5.2	2.6	✓	—	✓	✓	✓	✓	—	—
NC	—	—	11.6	17.9	✓	✓	✓	✓	—	✓	—	—
ND	—	—	3.2	2.7	✓	✓	✓	✓	—	—	—	—
OH	—	13.1	20.9	17.9	—	✓	✓	✓	—	✓	✓	—
OK	—	—	0.5	—	✓	✓	✓	✓	—	—	✓	—
OR	1.6	10.6	22.3	25.8	✓	✓	✓	✓	✓	—	✓	—
SC	—	—	2.7	2.4	✓	✓	✓	✓	—	—	—	—
UT	—	—	—	10.2	—	✓	✓	✓	✓	✓	—	—
VA	—	—	24.6	20.0	—	✓	✓	✓	—	—	—	✓
WA	7.9	20.7	19.0	12.0	✓	✓	✓	✓	✓	✓	—	✓
WI	—	23.4	33.3	23.3	—	✓	✓	✓	—	—	—	✓
WV	—	—	0.1	—	—	✓	✓	✓	✓	—	—	—

Note: Each of these outreach and enrollment efforts is described in the Commission's March 2011 Report to the Congress (pp. 68–69). Preliminary bonus payments may be revised to reflect final figures showing growth in children's enrollment in Medicaid.

[1] Originally, Alabama's bonus payments were $40 million for FY 2009 and $55 million for FY 2010. A preliminary audit conducted by CMS and the state revealed an error in the state's calculation of qualifying children. The FY 2009 and FY 2010 amounts in the table reflect the adjusted results from that preliminary audit.

Sources: U.S. Department of Health and Human Services (HHS), CHIPRA performance bonuses, December 2012, http://www.insurekidsnow.gov/professionals/eligibility/performance_bonuses.html, and MACPAC communication with Centers for Medicare & Medicaid Services, December 2012

MACStats

CHAPTER 4

Medicaid Coverage of Premiums and Cost Sharing for Low-Income Medicare Beneficiaries

Key Points

Medicaid Coverage of Premiums and Cost Sharing for Low-Income Medicare Beneficiaries

- For certain low-income beneficiaries, Medicaid pays for Medicare out-of-pocket costs such as premiums, coinsurance, and deductibles. Over time, Medicaid coverage of Medicare premiums and cost sharing has incrementally expanded. Today, there are four Medicare Savings Programs (MSPs), each with different income and asset level requirements:
    - qualified Medicare beneficiaries (QMBs),
    - specified low-income Medicare beneficiaries (SLMBs),
    - qualifying individuals (QIs), and
    - qualifying disabled and working individuals (QDWIs).

- In 2007, Medicaid payments for Medicare premiums totalled $10.5 billion, and Medicaid payments for acute care, which includes Medicare cost sharing and services not covered by Medicare, totalled $21.4 billion.

- Under current law, states have flexibility in how they pay providers for Medicare cost-sharing amounts. MACPAC's analysis shows that most states choose to limit their payment of Medicare deductibles and coinsurance to the lesser of the Medicare cost-sharing amount, or the difference between the Medicare payment and the Medicaid rate for the service.

- The study finds that Medicaid payment policies for Medicare cost sharing vary both among states and among the provider types examined within individual states, including:
    - about 40 states limit their payments for Medicare cost sharing for each of the services examined,
    - about half of the states limit payments for all examined provider types, and
    - only four states pay Medicare's full deductibles and coinsurance for every provider type.

- Medicare pays certain providers (e.g., hospitals, skilled nursing facilities) for a portion of the cost sharing that cannot be collected from beneficiaries (often referred to as bad debt). The cost sharing for dual eligibles that is not paid by state Medicaid agencies as a result of lesser-of policies is included in these Medicare bad debt payments.

- These Medicaid and Medicare policies can interact to shift costs between the two programs. These interactions also raise questions about the potential impact on access to care for beneficiaries whose Medicare cost sharing is paid by Medicaid.

CHAPTER 4

Medicaid Coverage of Premiums and Cost Sharing for Low-Income Medicare Beneficiaries

From its earliest days, Medicaid has contributed to the costs of medical care for low-income Medicare beneficiaries. Depending upon an individual's eligibility, this may include payment of Medicare premiums, coinsurance payments, and deductibles. It may also include full Medicaid coverage for services that are not covered by Medicare.

Unlike the Medicaid program, the Medicare program was originally designed to serve eligible individuals without regard to their income and included beneficiary cost-sharing requirements similar to private health insurance. While Medigap and employer-sponsored insurance plans provide supplemental coverage for many Medicare beneficiaries, low-income beneficiaries are less likely to have such coverage. Medicare's cost-sharing requirements may be a burden for people who live in poverty or have incomes just above poverty. For Medicare beneficiaries with incomes between 100 and 200 percent of the federal poverty level (FPL) in 2006, Medicare out-of-pocket spending accounted for nearly 25 percent of income (Nonnemaker and Sinclair 2011). Out of concern that low-income individuals would forgo needed care when faced with cost-sharing requirements beyond their means, the Congress made Medicaid's role in paying for these costs explicit over time through the creation of the Medicare Savings Programs (MSPs).

The MSPs, described in detail in the following sections, provided coverage for Medicare Part A and Part B cost-sharing expenses for 8.3 million out of a total of 10.2 million persons dually eligible for Medicaid and Medicare in 2011. Of these, 2.7 million Medicare beneficiaries received assistance only with cost sharing or premiums. Another 5.6 million individuals qualified for full Medicaid benefits and were also enrolled in one of the MSPs.

In 2007, Medicaid payments for Medicare premiums accounted for $10.5 billion, or 10 percent of Medicaid spending for all dual eligibles. Medicaid payments for acute care, which includes Medicare coinsurance and deductibles as well as other services not covered by Medicare, are estimated at $21.4 billion, or 20 percent of Medicaid spending for all dual eligibles in 2007.[1]

States have a certain amount of flexibility in how they pay for Medicare's cost sharing, but information on current state policies has not been readily available at the federal level. For this report, MACPAC reviewed state policies in order to develop an up-to-date and complete picture of how states pay for these cost-sharing amounts. The review shows that, as permitted under current law, most states choose to limit their payment of Medicare deductibles and coinsurance to the lesser of the cost-sharing amount, or the difference between the Medicare payment and the Medicaid rate for the service.[2]

The Commission is examining Medicaid coverage of Medicare premiums and cost sharing as part of its ongoing analytic agenda related to individuals who are dually eligible for Medicaid and Medicare, as well as its longstanding interest in Medicaid payment policy. It seeks to understand better the interaction between the Medicaid and Medicare programs at the state level, and, ultimately, whether such interactions affect access to services for dually eligible individuals. This chapter outlines Medicaid's coverage of Medicare premiums and cost sharing, including:

- an overview of the different programs that comprise the MSPs, including how state policies affect eligibility and enrollment of beneficiaries into these programs;
- results from a new MACPAC analysis that examines state Medicaid payment policies for Medicare cost sharing and discussion of the interaction with Medicare bad debt policy; and
- discussion of several policy questions related to Medicaid coverage of Medicare premiums and cost sharing.

Overview of Medicare Savings Programs

Since the programs' enactment in 1965, it has been possible for individuals to enroll in both Medicare and Medicaid if they are eligible for both programs, as described in Chapter 3 of this report. The Medicare program provides health insurance coverage to persons age 65 and over and persons with disabilities. Medicare Part A generally pays for institutional services such as hospital and skilled nursing facility (SNF) services, and Part B generally pays for outpatient services such as physician and laboratory services and durable medical equipment.[3] Both Part A and Part B services are subject to deductibles and coinsurance, and Part B also requires a monthly premium (Table 4-1).

Out of concern that Medicare's out-of-pocket costs could be a substantial burden for low-income Medicare beneficiaries who might not qualify for Medicaid in every state, possibly limiting access to necessary services, the Congress created programs to cover some of the costs. These programs use Medicaid as the mechanism to cover Medicare's costs, requiring states to "buy in" to the Medicare program for certain low-income Medicare beneficiaries by covering premiums and sometimes cost sharing. Medicare enrollees who meet the eligibility requirements for MSPs but have either too much income or too many assets to qualify for full Medicaid coverage in their state are often referred to as partial benefit dual eligibles.

Medicare Savings Programs

Over time, Medicaid coverage of Medicare premiums and cost sharing has incrementally

TABLE 4-1. Medicare Fee-for-Service Cost-Sharing Amounts for Part A and Part B Services, Calendar Year 2013[1]

	Part A	Part B
Premiums[2]	No premiums for most beneficiaries[3]	$104.90/month
Deductibles	Inpatient hospital: $1,184 Mental health inpatient: $1,184	$147/year
Copay/coinsurance	Durable medical equipment (DME) ▸ 20% of Medicare-approved amount for DME Inpatient hospital ▸ Days 61–90: $296/day ▸ Days 91+: $592/day for lifetime reserve days Mental health inpatient ▸ Days 61–90: $296/day ▸ Days 91+: $592/day for lifetime reserve days Nursing homes ▸ Days 21–100: $148/day ▸ Days 100+: all costs	Generally 20% of Medicare-approved amount

Notes:
1 Many of the cost-sharing amounts expressed as specific dollar amounts in this table are adjusted every year. For example, the Part B premium amounts are adjusted each year so that expected Medicare premium revenues equal 25 percent of expected Medicare Part B spending (42 U.S.C.§1395r(a)).
2 Medicare beneficiaries with incomes over $85,000 (or $170,000 for a couple) pay more for their premiums per month.
3 A Medicare beneficiary generally does not pay premiums for Medicare Part A unless the beneficiary or spouse has worked fewer than 40 quarters in his or her lifetime. For beneficiaries who do have to pay a Part A premium, it can be up to $441/month.

Source: CMS 2013b

---

expanded. Today, four different programs make up the MSPs, each with different qualifications based on an individual's income and assets:

▸ qualified Medicare beneficiaries (QMBs);
▸ specified low-income Medicare beneficiaries (SLMBs);
▸ qualifying individuals (QIs); and
▸ qualifying disabled and working individuals (QDWIs).

The first of the MSPs, the QMB program, was enacted in 1986 as a state option and then made mandatory in the Medicare Catastrophic Coverage Act of 1988 (MCAA, P.L. 110-360).[4] This law required states to cover all Medicare premiums and cost sharing for dual eligibles with incomes up to 100 percent FPL. The MSPs have been expanded over the years to additional low-income Medicare beneficiaries.

Table 4-2 highlights the four groups of MSP enrollees, including 2011 enrollment and 2013 eligibility and benefits. The following sections describe each group in more detail.

Qualified Medicare Beneficiary program (QMB). The QMB program is the first and most expansive of the MSPs in terms of the number of enrollees and benefits offered. (See Table 4-3 for this and other legislative milestones.) States

TABLE 4-2. Medicaid Benefits by Dual-Eligible Category

Dual Eligible Category	Medicaid Benefit Status	Enrollees in 2011 (millions)	Description	Federal Income Limits	2013 Federal Resource Limits (Individual/Couple)	Medicaid Benefits
Medicare Savings Programs (MSPs)						
Qualified Medicare beneficiaries (QMBs)	Partial benefit (QMB only)	1.3	Qualify for Medicaid payment of all Medicare premiums and cost sharing, but are otherwise ineligible for Medicaid in their state	Up to 100% FPL	$7,080/ $10,620	Medicare Part A premiums (if needed) Medicare Part B premiums Medicare deductibles and coinsurance
	Full benefit (QMB plus)	5.3	Qualify for Medicaid payment of all Medicare premiums and cost sharing, and also meet Medicaid eligibility criteria in their state and qualify for full Medicaid benefits	Up to 100% FPL	$2,000/ $3,000	Medicare Part A premiums (if needed) Medicare Part B premiums Medicare deductibles and coinsurance Full Medicaid benefits
Specified low-income Medicare beneficiaries (SLMBs)	Partial benefit (SLMB only)	0.9	Qualify for Medicaid payment of Medicare Part B premiums and are otherwise ineligible for Medicaid in their state	Between 100 and 120% FPL	$7,080/ $10,620	Medicare Part B premiums
	Full benefit (SLMB plus)	0.3	Qualify for Medicaid payment of Medicare Part B premiums, and also meet Medicaid eligibility criteria in their state and qualify for full Medicaid benefits, which includes payment for Medicare cost sharing within the limits of the state plan. Depending on their state, they may also receive Medicaid payment of Medicare Part A premiums.	Between 100 and 120% FPL	$2,000/ $3,000	Medicare Part B premiums Medicare deductibles and coinsurance (within the limits of the state plan) Medicare Part A premiums at state option Full Medicaid benefits

TABLE 4-2, Continued

Dual Eligible Category	Medicaid Benefit Status	Enrollees in 2011 (millions)	Description	Federal Income Limits	2013 Federal Resource Limits (Individual/Couple)	Medicaid Benefits
Qualified individuals (QIs)	Partial benefit	0.5	Qualify for Medicaid payment for Medicare Part B premiums and are otherwise ineligible for Medicaid in their state	Between 120 and 135% FPL	$7,080/ $10,620	Medicare Part B premiums
Qualified disabled and working individuals (QDWIs)	Partial benefit	Fewer than 100 individuals	Have lost their Medicare Part A benefits due to their return to work but are eligible to purchase Medicare Part A, qualify for Medicaid payment of Medicare Part A premiums, and are otherwise ineligible for Medicaid in their state.	At or below 200% FPL	$4,000/ $6,000	Medicare Part A premiums
Non-MSP						
Other full-benefit dual eligibles	Full benefit	1.9	Do not meet income or resource requirements for QMB, SLMB, or QI but meet Medicaid eligibility criteria in their state and qualify for full Medicaid benefits, which includes payment for Medicare cost sharing covered within the limits of the state plan. Depending on their state they may also receive Medicaid payment of Medicare Part A premiums.	Varies by state and Medicaid eligibility pathway	$2,000/ $3,000	Full Medicaid benefits Medicare coinsurance and deductibles (within the limits of the state plan) Medicare Part A premiums at state option

Notes: FPL is the federal poverty level. Section 1902(r)(2) of the Social Security Act allows states to use income and resource methodologies that are "less restrictive," enabling states to expand eligibility above these standards. Not all resources (e.g., value of house, value of one vehicle, etc.) are counted toward resource limits. Section 209(b) states may use Medicaid eligibility criteria that are more restrictive than the Supplemental Security Income program, but may not use more restrictive criteria than those in effect in the state on January 1, 1972. For information on state Medicaid income eligibility levels for persons age 65 and over and individuals with disabilities, see MACStats Table 11. Resource limits for QMB, SLMB, and QI are adjusted annually for inflation. QI expenditures are fully federally funded and total expenditures are limited by statute. Medicaid coverage of additional premiums for Medicare Advantage plans is optional for states (§1905(p)(3)(D)).

Source: Enrollees in 2011: CMS 2013a; Description and Federal Income Limits: §1902(a)(10)(E) of the Social Security Act; 2013 Federal Resource Limits: SSA 2012

are required to cover Medicare Part B premiums and all Medicare deductibles and coinsurance for Medicare beneficiaries with incomes up to 100 percent FPL ($11,490 for an individual and $4,020 for each additional family member in 2013).[5] Medicaid spending for Medicare premiums, deductibles, and coinsurance is eligible for federal financial participation (FFP).

All Medicare beneficiaries with incomes up to 100 percent FPL and assets under $7,080 for an individual in fiscal year (FY) 2013 are eligible for the QMB program, regardless of whether or not they qualify for full Medicaid benefits in their state. There are two types of QMBs. Just over 20 percent of QMBs do not otherwise qualify for full Medicaid benefits (these individuals are known as "QMB-only" dual eligibles). Medicaid coverage for QMB-only dual eligibles is limited to Medicare premiums and cost sharing. The other 80 percent consists of beneficiaries—such as Supplemental Security Income (SSI) recipients and certain medically needy individuals—who meet the QMB criteria and are also eligible for full Medicaid benefits in their state (commonly known as "QMB-plus" dual eligibles). In addition to Medicaid coverage of Medicare premiums and cost sharing, these QMB-plus individuals receive full Medicaid benefits, including some—such as long-term services and supports (LTSS), dental, and vision—that are not covered in the Medicare program.

Specified Low-income Medicare Beneficiary program (SLMB). The Omnibus Budget and Reconciliation Act of 1990 (OBRA 90, P.L. 101-508) expanded Medicaid coverage of Medicare Part B premiums to Medicare beneficiaries with incomes between 100 and 120 percent FPL (120 percent FPL is $13,788 for an individual and $4,824 for each additional family member in 2013). Medicaid payments for Part B premiums are eligible for FFP. This incremental expansion was a result of efforts by the Congress to mitigate the effect on low-income Medicare beneficiaries of provisions in OBRA 90 that increased Medicare Part B premiums (Committee on the Budget 1990).

All Medicare beneficiaries with incomes between 100 and 120 percent FPL are eligible for the SLMB program, regardless of their eligibility for full Medicaid benefits. As with QMBs, there are some SLMBs that receive full Medicaid benefits (SLMB-plus dual eligibles), generally through a medically needy eligibility pathway. There are also SLMBs who do not qualify for full Medicaid benefits in their state and who receive Medicaid coverage for only their Part B premiums (SLMB-only dual eligibles). The SLMB program, like the QMB program, is an entitlement with no caps on enrollment or spending. In 2011 there were around 900,000 dual eligibles enrolled as SLMB-only dual eligibles and around 300,000 enrolled as SLMB-plus dual eligibles.

Qualifying Individual program (QI). The Balanced Budget Act of 1997 (BBA, P.L. 105-33) further expanded Medicaid coverage of Medicare Part B premiums to Medicare beneficiaries with incomes between 120 and 135 percent FPL (QIs). Unlike the QMB and SLMB programs, the QI program is a limited entitlement that is based on a specific allotment of funds to each state. QI funds are allocated to states in one-year increments, based on congressional appropriations and periodic reauthorizations of the program.[6]

State payments for Part B premiums on behalf of QIs are fully funded by the federal government, subject to state-specific limits. If a state surpasses the amount allocated, then the state is fully responsible for the remaining expenses. Federal statute permits states to impose restrictions on enrollment policies for QIs, including limiting the number of QIs in a given year. Enrollment in the QI program is typically on a first-come, first-served basis, and each enrollee must re-apply to the QI program every year (§1933(b) of the Social Security Act (the Act)). In 2011 there were around 500,000 dual eligibles enrolled in the QI program.

Qualifying Disabled and Working Individual program (QDWI). A fourth program to provide Medicaid coverage of Medicare Part A premiums was implemented as a result of the Omnibus Budget and Reconciliation Act of 1989 (OBRA 89, P.L. 101-239), which included changes in the Medicare law intended to help individuals with disabilities retain Medicare coverage. Before OBRA 89, many individuals with disabilities could lose their Medicare Part A and Social Security coverage (i.e., Social Security Disability Insurance) as a result of returning to work. Their relatively high need for health care services made it difficult for this group of working individuals with disabilities to purchase private health insurance. This also served as a disincentive for some employers, particularly smaller employers, to hire individuals with disabilities due to the effect they might have on the employers' group health insurance premiums.

OBRA 89 allowed persons with disabilities whose work activities caused them to lose Medicare and Social Security to purchase Medicare Part A and Part B coverage. Furthermore, the law mandated that state Medicaid programs cover the Medicare Part A premiums for individuals in this category who have incomes below 200 percent FPL and resources not in excess of twice the SSI resource levels ($4,000 for an individual and $6,000 for a couple). In 2011 there were fewer than 100 beneficiaries enrolled as QDWIs.

Non-MSP full-benefit dual eligibles. There are also individuals who are eligible for both Medicaid and Medicare but not for the MSP programs. Non-MSP full-benefit dual eligibles are generally individuals who spend down to qualify as medically needy in Medicaid, or who meet special income levels and are institutionalized or enrolled in home and community-based waivers. While these individuals receive full Medicaid benefits in accordance with each state's Medicaid state plan, there is no statutory requirement for Medicaid coverage of Medicare coinsurance and deductibles as there is for QMBs. States may choose, however, to cover these amounts as cost sharing, or as coverage of the underlying service according to their state plan. States also have the option of covering non-MSP dual eligibles' Part B premiums.[7] In 2011 there were about 2 million non-MSP full-benefit dual eligibles.

Role of States in Medicare Savings Program Eligibility and Enrollment

State Medicaid agencies administer the MSPs, and therefore play a significant role in determining eligibility and benefits, as well as other policies and procedures that can affect the rate of enrollment in the programs. While federal requirements establish a baseline for MSP eligibility, states have flexibility to increase eligibility by using different methods for determining income and resources. As a result, the number of MSP enrollees varies across states. Enrollment rates in the MSPs have generally been low, however, compared to the number of individuals who are estimated to be eligible for the programs (CBO 2004).

Eligibility

Federal standards for counting income and resources for MSP eligibility were initially based on those used by the federal SSI program. Before

TABLE 4-3. Legislative Milestones in Medicaid Coverage of Premiums and Cost Sharing for Low-Income Medicare Beneficiaries

1965 The Medicare program was enacted as Title XVIII of the Social Security Act of 1965 (P.L. 89–97) to provide health care coverage for individuals age 65 and older. The Medicaid program was enacted as Title XIX of the Social Security Act to provide health coverage for low-income individuals, including coverage for low-income Medicare beneficiaries (dual eligibles).
- For low-income individuals entitled to both Medicare and Medicaid, states were given the option to either pay for these individuals' Part B services directly as a Medicaid service (eligible for federal match) or states could pay the Medicare Part B premium and Medicare would be the primary payer of the covered services.

1967 The Social Security Amendments of 1967 (P.L. 90–248) prohibited federal financial participation for Medicaid services that could have been paid for by Medicare Part B if the recipient had been enrolled.

1986 The Omnibus Budget Reconciliation Act of 1986 (P.L. 99–509) permitted states to provide Medicaid benefits to low-income qualified Medicare beneficiaries (QMBs) with incomes at or below 100 percent of the federal poverty level (FPL). States had the option to provide either of two Medicaid benefit packages:
- Limit coverage to Medicare premiums and cost sharing or
- Provide full Medicaid benefits in addition to Medicare premiums and cost sharing.

1988 The Medicare Catastrophic Coverage Act of 1988 (MCCA, P.L. 100–360) enacted provisions that required states to cover QMBs but limited the Medicaid benefits to Medicare premiums and cost sharing. This was the first of the programs now commonly referred to as the Medicare Savings Programs (MSPs). Most of the MCCA was repealed in 1989, but the MSP requirements for QMB coverage remained in law.

1989 The Omnibus Budget Reconciliation Act of 1989 (P.L. 101–239)
- Established a new eligibility group for disabled and working individuals—those who previously qualified for Medicare because of disability but lost their Medicare coverage because of their return to work—who may purchase Medicare Part A and Part B coverage. States are required to pay the Medicare Part A premiums for these individuals with incomes below 200 percent FPL (known as qualified disabled and working individuals (QDWIs)). This was the second of the programs now known as MSPs.
- Prohibited providers from balance billing dual eligibles (i.e., when a provider sends the beneficiary a bill that exceeds the beneficiary share of the Medicare rate for the service).

1990 The Omnibus Budget Reconciliation Act of 1990 (P.L. 101–508) required states to pay Medicare Part B premiums for beneficiaries with incomes between 100 and 120 percent FPL (special low-income Medicare beneficiaries (SLMBs)). This was the third MSP.

TABLE 4-3, Continued

1997   The Balanced Budget Act of 1997 (P.L. 105–33)
- Required states to pay Medicare Part B premiums for Medicare beneficiaries with incomes between 120 and 135 percent FPL (qualifying individuals (QIs)), the fourth MSP. This benefit is subject to an annual federal funding cap that limits the number of QIs served in a given year.
- Stated that state Medicaid programs may limit their payment for Medicare cost sharing for QMBs to the difference between the state's Medicaid rate and the Medicare payment amount as long as their payment policies are written in their state plan.
- Prohibited Medicare providers or Medicare managed care entities from directly charging any Medicare cost sharing directly to QMBs. They must consider the amount paid by the state for Medicare cost sharing to be payment in full for any QMBs that they serve.

2003   The Medicare Prescription Drug, Improvement, and Modernization Act of 2003 (P.L. 108–173) established a voluntary outpatient prescription drug benefit for people on Medicare, known as Part D, that went into effect January 1, 2006.
- Changed prescription drug coverage for individuals dually eligible for Medicare and Medicaid from Medicaid to private Medicare Part D plans.
- Provided the low-income subsidy (LIS), an additional subsidy for beneficiaries with limited assets and income to help pay a portion of out-of-pocket prescription drug costs. Medicare beneficiaries who receive the LIS often qualify for the subsidy automatically on the basis of being Medicaid or Supplemental Security Income (SSI) recipients, or because they are enrolled in certain MSPs.

2008   The Medicare Improvements for Patients and Providers Act of 2008 (P.L. 110–275)
- Increased the federal asset limits for MSPs (which had previously been frozen at $4,000 for an individual and $6,000 for couples) to the same level as the full Part D LIS asset limits and indexed to inflation thereafter. This change took effect January 1, 2010.
- Required the Social Security Administration to transfer information from an LIS application to the state Medicaid agency, which is required to use it to initiate an application for MSP enrollment.

2010   The Patient Protection and Affordable Care Act (P.L. 111–148)
- Created the Federal Coordinated Health Care Office (FCHCO) in the Centers for Medicare & Medicaid Services to explore methods of aligning and coordinating benefits between the Medicaid and Medicare programs more effectively and efficiently. The FCHCO is partnering with states and plans to test the alignment of service delivery and financing between the programs through the financial alignment demonstration.
- Eliminated Part D cost sharing for full-benefit dual-eligible beneficiaries receiving home and community-based services who would otherwise require institutional care (beneficiaries residing in institutional settings already had no cost sharing).
- Prohibited Medicare Advantage plans and their providers from directly charging dual eligibles for Medicare Part A and Part B cost sharing.

the passage of the Medicare Improvements for Patients and Providers Act of 2008 (MIPPA, P.L. 110-275), the federal resource limit for MSPs had not been raised since the QMB program was enacted in 1988 (GAO 2012). Beginning in 2010, the federal resource limits for all MSPs were uniformly tied to the resource limits of the Medicare Part D low-income subsidy (LIS) program, to be adjusted for inflation in the future. In 2013, the resource limits for the QMB, SLMB, QI, and LIS programs are $7,080 for an individual and $10,620 for a couple (SSA 2012). However, states are permitted to disregard amounts of income or resources when determining MSP eligibility, effectively increasing the number of individuals that can qualify. In 2006, 39 states used one or more methods to count income and resources that result in limits that are higher than the federal standards (Nemore 2006).

States also have flexibility in determining eligibility for full Medicaid benefits, including for full-benefit dual eligibles (see Chapter 3 and MACStats Table 11). This variability in eligibility means that Medicare beneficiaries with the same income and resources are eligible for different benefits in different states. For example, in one state, an individual may qualify as a QMB-plus dual eligible and, therefore, receive full Medicaid benefits in addition to Medicare cost sharing. In another state the same beneficiary could be eligible as a QMB-only dual eligible, entitled only to Medicaid coverage of Medicare cost sharing.

Enrollment

Historically, MSP enrollment rates among eligible Medicare beneficiaries have been low. In 2004, the Congressional Budget Office estimated that 33 percent of eligible beneficiaries were enrolled in QMB programs and only 13 percent of eligible individuals were enrolled in SLMB programs (CBO 2004).[8] A 2002 study estimated that fewer than 19 percent of eligible beneficiaries were enrolled as QIs (Summer and Friedland 2002).

Beneficiaries' lack of awareness about the programs and complex eligibility and enrollment processes are cited as primary barriers to enrollment in MSPs (Haber et al. 2003, Glaun 2002, Neumann et al. 1994). Several MIPPA provisions aimed at eliminating barriers to MSP enrollment, such as aligning resource levels with those used for LIS and additional funding for states to perform outreach for MSPs, resulted in growth in the MSP enrollment rate in each year from FY 2007 through 2011 (GAO 2012).

Enrollment rates among those eligible for MSPs have been shown to vary across states (Rosenbach and Lamphere 1999). States face conflicting incentives for increasing enrollment in their MSPs. On one hand, the programs may improve access to care for Medicare beneficiaries with low incomes. On the other hand, for QMBs, SLMBs, and QDWIs, increasing the number of beneficiaries enrolled will result in increased Medicaid expenditures. The varying rates of enrollment into the MSPs may depend on a state's eligibility and outreach activities. For example, enrollment in the QMB and SLMB programs in states that participated in the Robert Wood Johnson Foundation's State Solutions grant program increased 45 percent from 2002 to 2005, compared to a 22 percent increase nationwide during that same time period (Summer 2006). Strategies included modifying eligibility requirements, expanding outreach activities, simplifying the enrollment process, training staff and volunteers to conduct enrollment activities, and strengthening data collection.

States' Role in Determining Payment for Medicare Coinsurance and Deductibles

State flexibility in Medicaid coverage of Medicare cost sharing extends to the amounts that states pay for Medicare coinsurance and deductibles. Claims for coinsurance and deductibles are commonly referred to as crossover claims, because providers first submit a claim to the Medicare program, which pays the provider for the service, and the claim then crosses over to Medicaid for payment of cost-sharing amounts.

States are not obligated to pay the full amount of Medicare coinsurance and deductibles if total payment to the provider would exceed the state's Medicaid rate. Instead, states may limit their payment through lesser-of policies that pay the lesser of:

- the full amount of Medicare deductibles and coinsurance; or
- the difference between the Medicaid rate and the amount already paid by Medicare (Box 4-1).

The following section describes the history of lesser-of policies as well as the results of a MACPAC survey of state payment policies for Medicare cost sharing. It also describes the interaction of state payment policies and Medicare bad debt payment and limitations in data regarding Medicaid payment of Medicare cost sharing.

History of lesser-of payment policies

The origin of the lesser-of policy can be traced to the enactment of the QMB program in 1988. While the legislation required state Medicaid programs to pay for QMBs' Medicare cost sharing, it did not specify whether states were obligated to pay providers the full amount, or only up to the state Medicaid rate (§1902(a)(10)(E)(i) of the Act). In an amendment to the State Medicaid Manual, the Health Care Financing Administration (HCFA, now CMS) allowed lesser-of policies (HCFA 1991). However, providers brought lawsuits in multiple jurisdictions arguing that the HCFA guidance, and state policies implementing lesser-of policies, did not fulfill the legal requirement that a state cover Medicare's cost sharing for QMBs. Federal court decisions on this question were mixed, with four courts finding that states must pay Medicare's full cost-sharing amounts and two upholding HCFA's policy (Waxman et al. 1997).

To resolve the uncertainty, in 1997 the BBA gave states explicit authority to use lesser-of policies (§4714 of the BBA, amending §1902(n) of the Act). States were required to file an amendment to their state plan (via Supplement 1 to Attachment 4.19-B) in order to specify their policy on payment of Medicare cost sharing (HCFA 1997). The BBA also clarified that providers cannot directly bill QMBs for any Medicare cost sharing, even if Medicaid does not pay the full amount. Instead, providers must accept payment from Medicare and Medicaid as payment in full.[9]

Medicaid payment of Medicare cost sharing for non-QMB full-benefit dual eligibles is not a statutorily required benefit. The Centers for Medicare & Medicaid Services (CMS) has indicated, however, that states may choose to treat Medicare cost sharing for these individuals as either: (1) coverage of the underlying service in accordance with the Medicaid state plan, or (2) coverage of cost sharing. Under the first option, Medicaid payment to a provider is the Medicaid rate for the service according to the state plan, minus any amount paid by Medicare or other payers. Because the Medicaid payment in this case is payment for a covered service (rather than for cost sharing), any income that an enrollee may be required to contribute toward Medicaid services

BOX 4-1. Examples of Medicaid Payment for Medicare Cost Sharing

The table below illustrates Medicaid payment of cost sharing for a service with a Medicare-approved amount of $100, when the state's Medicaid-approved rate for the same service is $90. If Medicare's payment is 80 percent of the approved amount, Medicare pays the provider $80, less any remaining deductible. The remaining 20 percent (in this case, $20), plus the amount of deductible applied, is billed to Medicaid as a crossover claim.

Full-payment policy. Some states pay the Medicare cost-sharing amount in full, regardless of what their Medicaid rate is for the service. In this example, the Medicaid payment from a state with a full payment policy would bring the total provider payment to $100.

Lesser-of policy. A state with a lesser-of policy would compare the requested Medicare cost sharing to the difference between the state's Medicaid rate and the Medicare payment amount, and pay the lesser amount. In this example, the Medicaid payment would bring the total amount paid to the provider to $90 (the Medicaid-approved rate).

In instances when Medicare has already paid more than the Medicaid rate for a particular service, under a lesser-of policy, Medicaid is not required to pay anything additional. For example, if Medicare pays $80 on the $100 claim, but Medicaid's rate for the service is only $70, then Medicaid will make no additional payment, and the claim is considered paid in full.

	Full-Payment Policy		Lesser-of Policy	
	Deductible not met	After deductible is met	Deductible not met	After deductible is met
Provider charge	$125	$125	$125	$125
Medicare-approved amount	$100	$100	$100	$100
Medicaid payment rate	$90	$90	$90	$90
Beneficiary's remaining Medicare deductible	$147	$0	$147	$0
Medicare payment (e.g., for physicians, 80% of Medicare-approved amount, minus deductible)	(80% of $100) − $147 = $0	(80% of $100) − $0 = $80	(80% of $100) − $147 = $0	(80% of $100) − $0 = $80
Medicare cost sharing (billed to Medicaid as a crossover claim)	$100	$20	$100	$20
Medicaid payment to provider	$100	$20	Lesser of Medicare cost sharing ($100) or Medicaid rate minus Medicare payment ($90−$0) = $90	Lesser of Medicare cost sharing ($20) or Medicaid rate minus Medicare payment ($90−$80) = $10

would be applied.[10] Under the second option, states may choose whether to limit payment of the Medicare cost sharing in the same manner as for QMBs, and enrollee income would not be applied (CMS 2012a).

For dual eligibles that are enrolled in Medicare managed care plans, state Medicaid agencies are still responsible for payment of deductibles and coinsurance. In some cases, states opt to contract with the Medicare managed care plan to cover the cost sharing on their behalf.[11] If the state does not contract with a plan to cover cost sharing, providers must be able to submit crossover claims directly to the state Medicaid program (CMS 2012b). Similarly, when dual eligibles are enrolled in Medicaid managed care plans, states may include an amount for Medicare cost sharing in the capitation rate paid to the plan, or may require providers to bill the state directly.

Inventory of State Medicaid Payment Policies for Medicare Coinsurance and Deductibles

Because the most recent information regarding individual state payment policies for deductibles and coinsurance was over 10 years old, MACPAC undertook a study of current policies in the 50 states and the District of Columbia. The study looked at crossover payment policies for four provider types: inpatient hospitals, outpatient hospitals, SNFs, and physicians, and classified each state's policy for each provider type as one of following three options:

▸ **Full payment:** The state pays the full amount of Medicare deductibles and coinsurance, so that the provider receives the full Medicare-approved amount.

▸ **Lesser of:** The state pays the lesser of two amounts: (1) the full Medicare deductible and coinsurance, or (2) the difference between the Medicaid rate and the amount already paid by Medicare.

▸ **Other:** The state payment policy does not clearly fall into either of the above categories (e.g., the state always pays a fixed percentage of the deductible and coinsurance).

We used publicly available materials to identify crossover payment policies for most states for four categories of Medicare services, then followed up with state staff to resolve any outstanding questions. Because Medicaid state plans are not always readily available, the study team focused on state regulations and provider manuals that were believed to reflect actual current practice. This decision was reinforced by recent Office of Inspector General (OIG) reports showing that some states' crossover policies did not follow what was approved in their state plan (OIG 2012a, 2012b, 2012c). In these cases, the OIG reported that the states paid the full amount of Medicare crossover claims for dual eligibles while their state plans indicated lesser-of policies.

Results by provider type. State Medicaid programs are much more likely to use lesser-of policies than to pay the full amount of Medicare coinsurance and deductibles (Figure 4-1). In a few cases, researchers classified payment policies as "other." For example:

▸ **Ratio of costs to charges.** Two states that pay hospitals on the basis of a ratio of costs to charges have chosen to apply that ratio to crossover claims rather than calculating a Medicaid-allowed amount and then a lesser-of amount for each service.

▸ **Percentage of Medicare's cost sharing.** Several states set a specific percentage of a

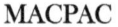

FIGURE 4-1. Number of Medicaid Programs Using Lesser-of, Full-Payment, and Other Crossover Policies, 2012

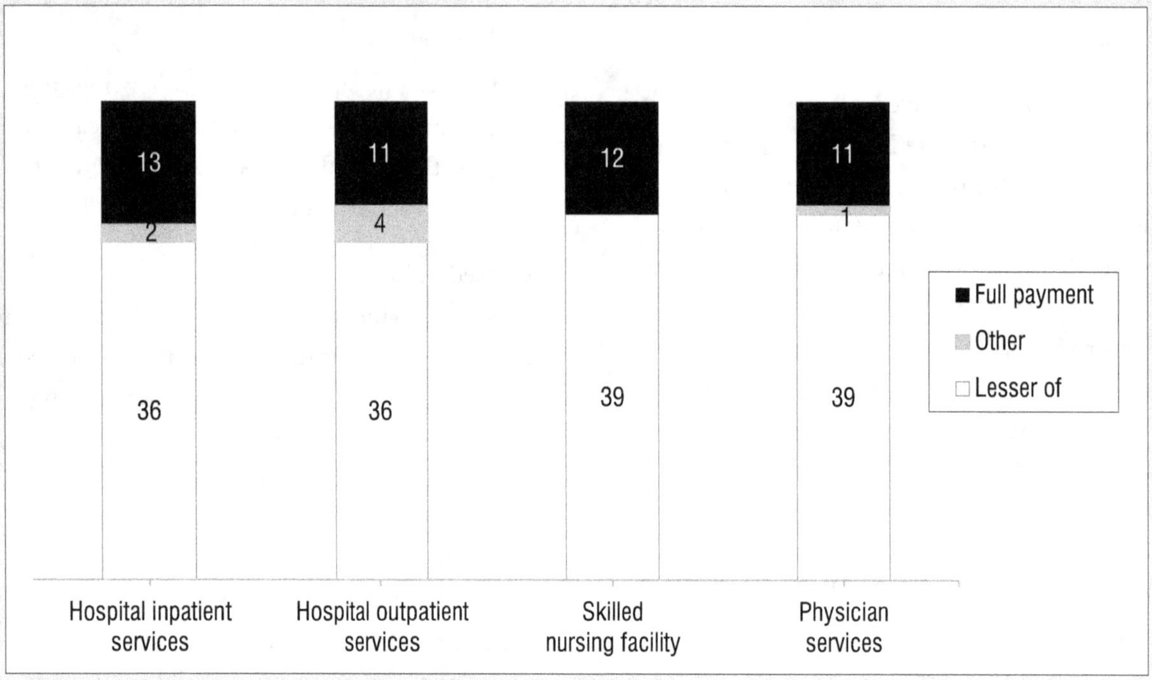

	Hospital inpatient services	Hospital outpatient services	Skilled nursing facility	Physician services
Full payment	13	11	12	11
Other	2	4	—	1
Lesser of	36	36	39	39

Source: Data collected by NORC at the University of Chicago for MACPAC.

Medicare crossover claim that they will pay, presumably as an estimate of an amount that is at least as much as they would pay under a lesser-of policy for the same type of provider.

Results within states. Crossover policies vary both among states and among provider types within individual states (Table 4-4 and Figures 4-2 to 4-5). Of the 51 Medicaid programs for which researchers collected information, about half have a lesser-of policy for all provider types. Only four states (Arkansas, Iowa, Vermont, and Wyoming) pay Medicare's full deductibles and coinsurance for every provider type that researchers investigated.

The remaining 18 states mix and match policies in almost every possible combination, with no clear patterns emerging. For example, Idaho and Montana pay the full amount for hospital inpatient and outpatient crossover claims, but use a lesser-of policy for SNFs and physicians. Hawaii does exactly the opposite, paying with a lesser-of policy for hospital-based services but paying the full amount for Medicare SNF and physician crossover claims.

Changes in crossover payment policies. From the limited information available, it appears that there has been a substantial shift toward lesser-of policies over time (Figure 4-6). Two surveys sought to track state Medicaid policies in the context of implementation of the BBA in the late 1990s. They both used a different methodology from the study conducted by MACPAC and did not differentiate among provider types. In the 1997

TABLE 4-4. Lesser-of, Full-Payment, and Other Crossover Policies, by State, 2012

	Inpatient	Outpatient	SNF	Physician		Inpatient	Outpatient	SNF	Physician
AK	L	L	L	L	MT	F	F	L	L
AL	F	L	F	L	NC	L	L	L	L
AR	F	F	F	F	ND	L	L	L	L
AZ	L	L	L	L	NE	F	F	L	F
CA	L	L	L	L	NH	L	L	L	L
CO	L	L	L	L	NJ	F	F	F	L
CT	L	L	L	L	NM	L	L	L	L
DC	L	L	L	L	NV	L	L	L	L
DE	F	L	F	L	NY	F	L	F	O
FL	L	L	L	L	OH	L	L	L	L
GA	L	O	L	L	OK	O	O	L	F
HI	L	L	F	F	OR	L	L	L	L
IA	F	F	F	F	PA	L	L	L	L
ID	F	F	L	L	RI	O	O	F	L
IL	L	L	L	L	SC	L	L	L	L
IN	L	L	L	L	SD	L	F	F	F
KS	L	L	L	L	TN	L	L	L	L
KY	L	F	L	L	TX	L	L	L	L
LA	L	L	L	L	UT	L	L	L	L
MA	L	L	L	L	VA	L	L	L	L
MD	F*	L	L	L	VT	F	F	F	F
ME	L	L	L	F	WA	L	L	L	L
MI	L	L	L	L	WI	L	L	F	L
MN	L	L	L	L	WV	L	L	L	L
MO	L	O	L	F	WY	F	F	F	F
MS	F	F	L	F					

Notes: SNF is skilled nursing facility. L is lesser of. F is full payment. O is other (i.e., not clearly lesser of nor full payment).
* Because of its all-payer waiver, Maryland's Medicaid and Medicare rates are the same for inpatient hospital services.
Source: Data collected by NORC at the University of Chicago for MACPAC. State-specific payment policy details and sources can be found at www.macpac.gov

MACPAC | REPORT TO THE CONGRESS ON MEDICAID AND CHIP

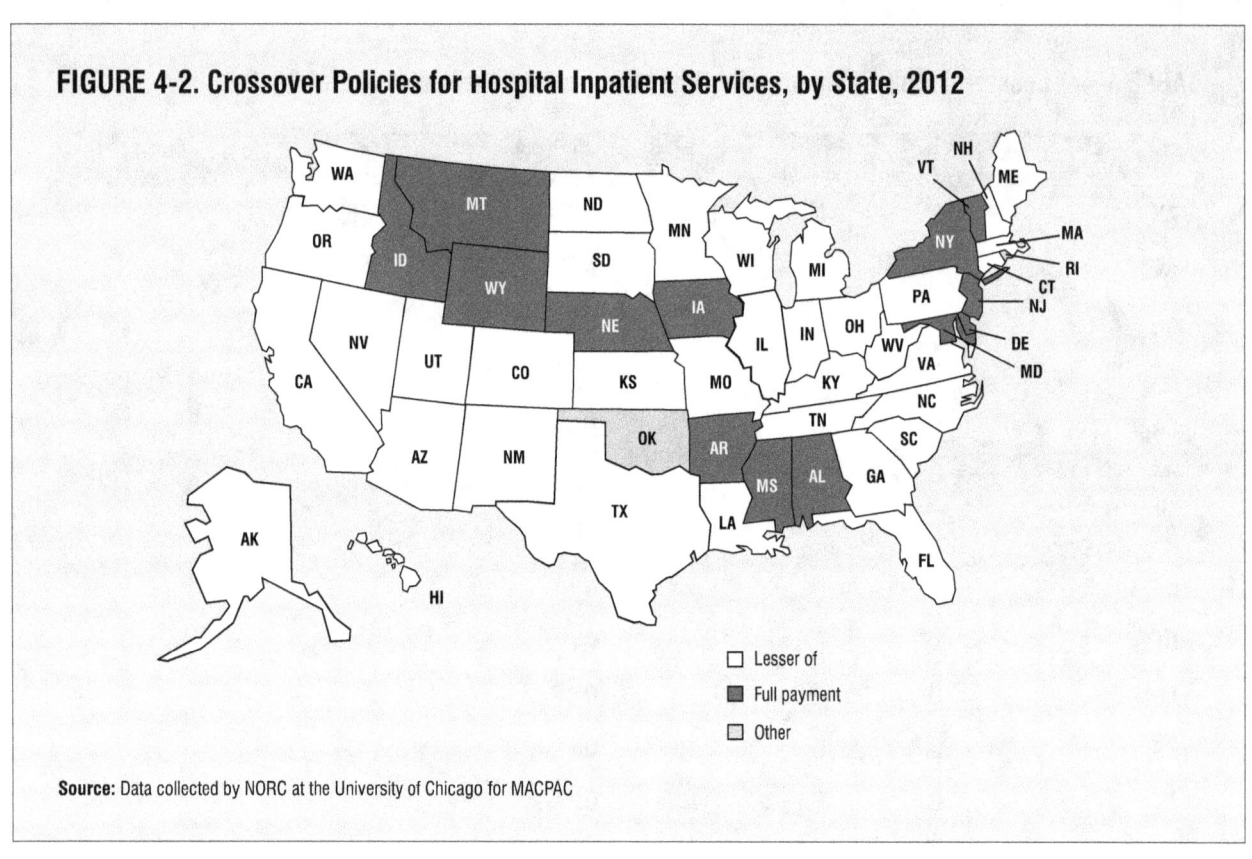

FIGURE 4-2. Crossover Policies for Hospital Inpatient Services, by State, 2012

Source: Data collected by NORC at the University of Chicago for MACPAC

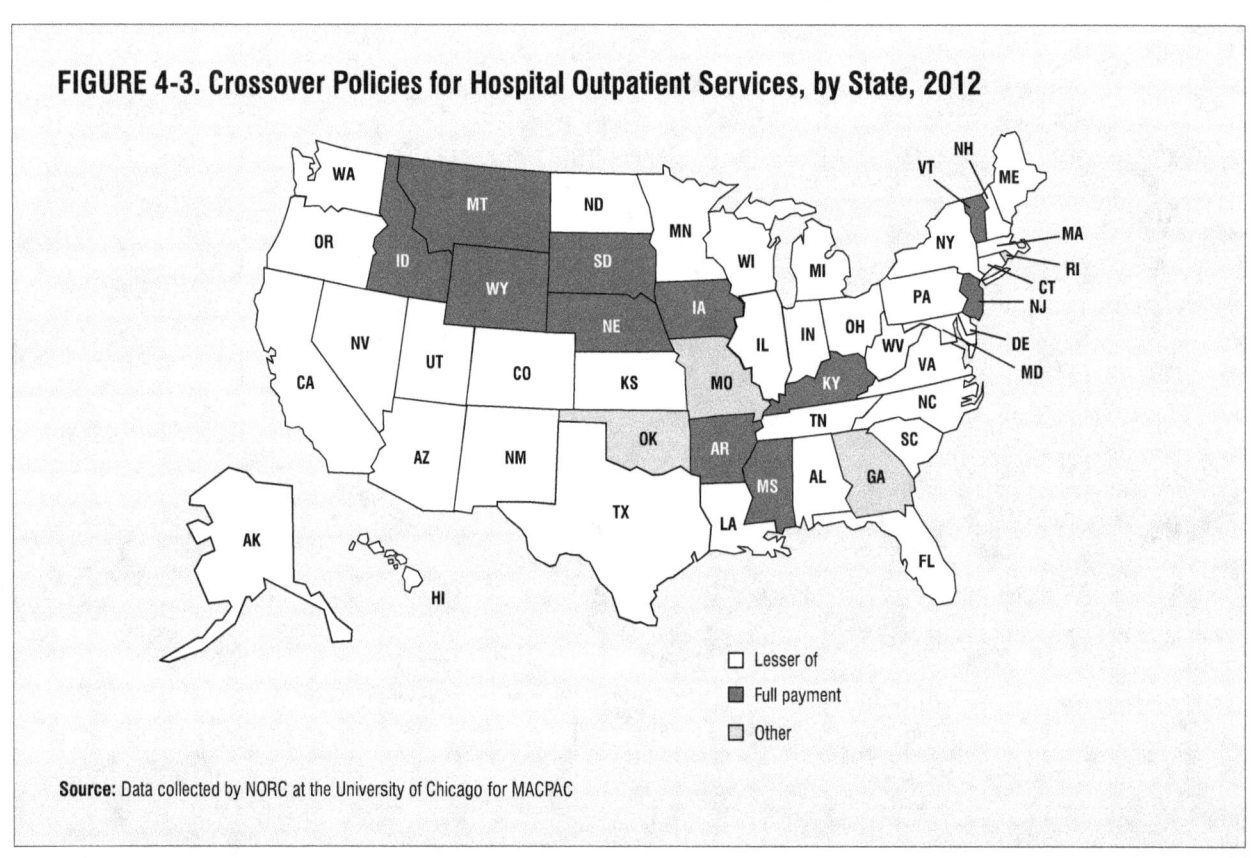

FIGURE 4-3. Crossover Policies for Hospital Outpatient Services, by State, 2012

Source: Data collected by NORC at the University of Chicago for MACPAC

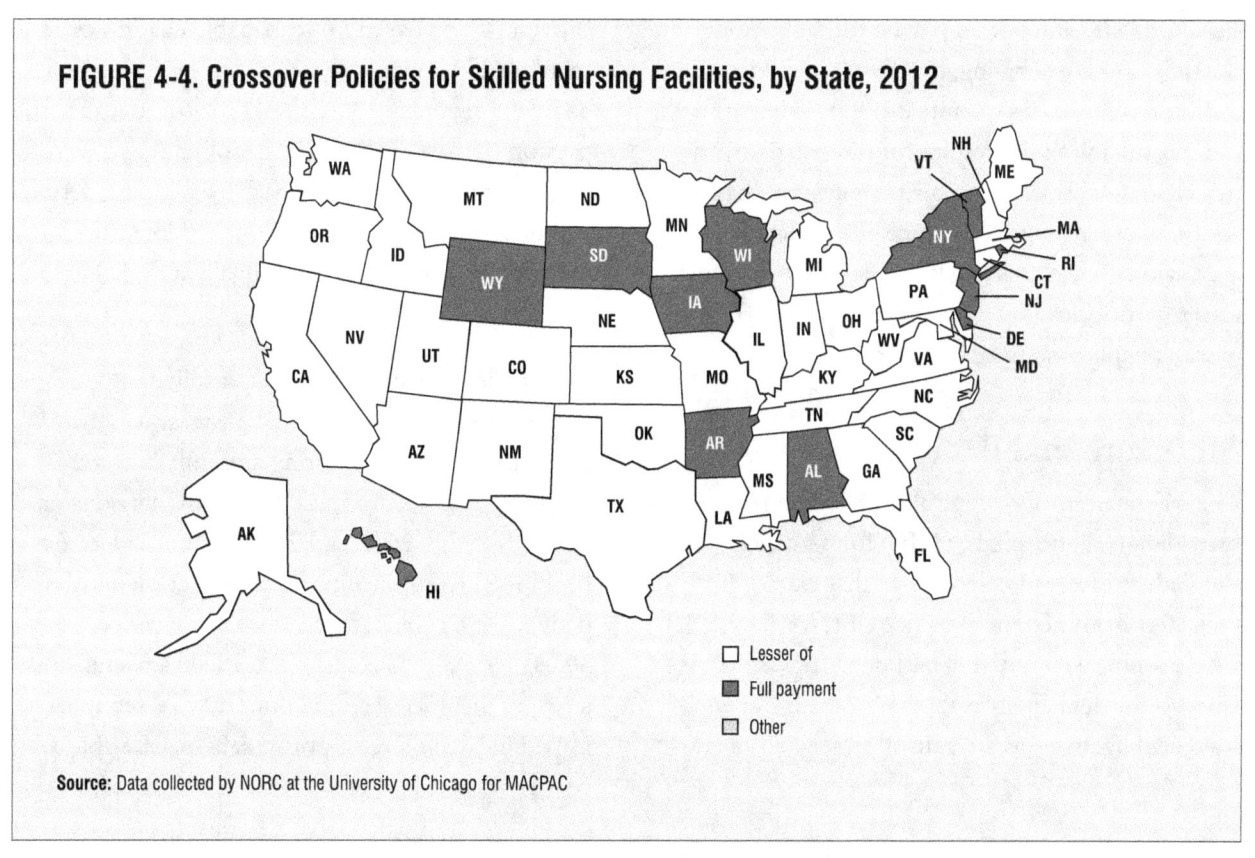

FIGURE 4-4. Crossover Policies for Skilled Nursing Facilities, by State, 2012

Source: Data collected by NORC at the University of Chicago for MACPAC

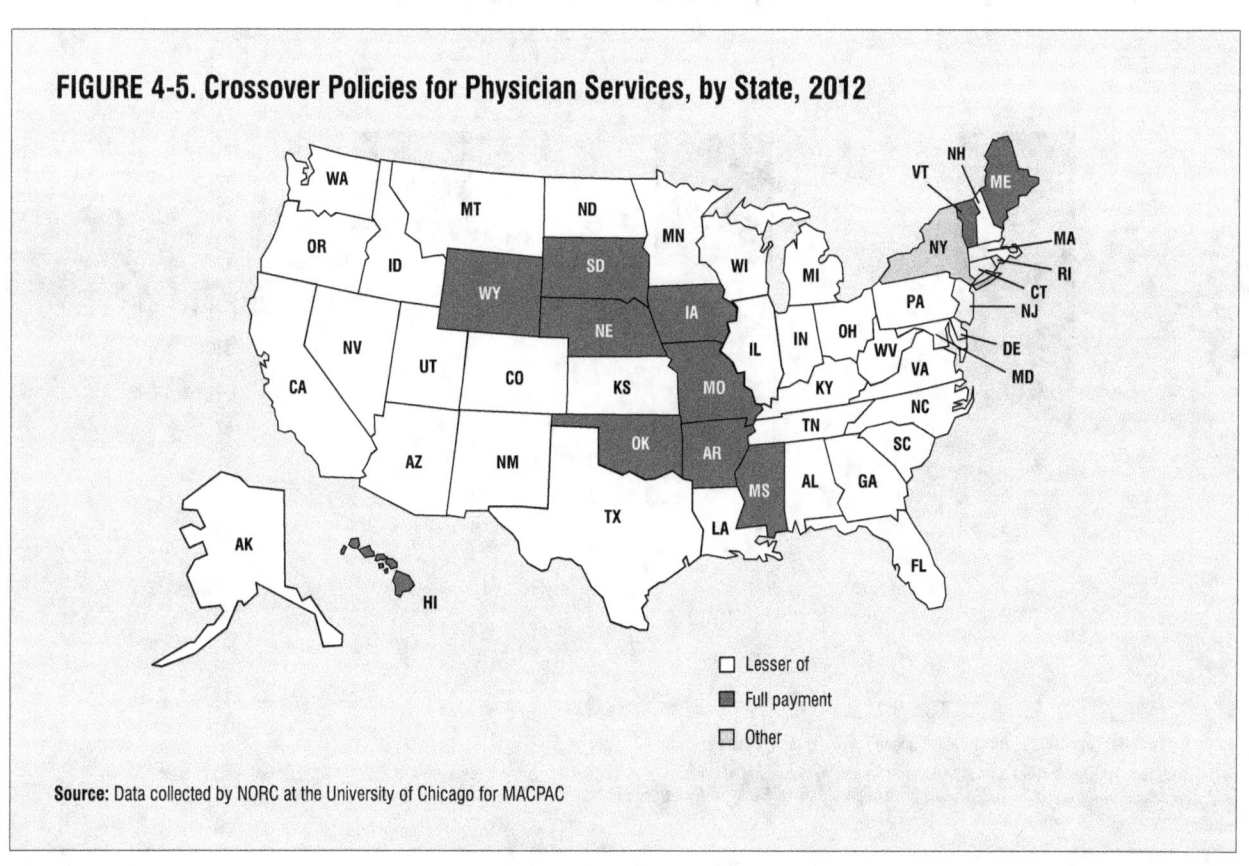

FIGURE 4-5. Crossover Policies for Physician Services, by State, 2012

Source: Data collected by NORC at the University of Chicago for MACPAC

survey, 31 states reported paying the full amount of Medicare cost sharing; by 1999, the number had dropped to 15 states (Nemore 1999). Comparing these results with the results for physicians from this report, it appears that additional states have adopted lesser-of policies since 1999. However, the majority of states appear to have adopted their lesser-of policies in the two years after the BBA granted explicit statutory authority.

Medicare bad debt payment

The Medicare program reimburses certain providers (e.g., hospitals, SNFs) for a portion of the deductibles and coinsurance that cannot be collected from beneficiaries (42 CFR §413.89). These amounts, known as bad debt, include cost sharing for dual eligibles that is not paid by state Medicaid agencies as a result of lesser-of policies.[12]

Providers paid based on reasonable charges or fee schedules, including physicians, are not eligible for bad debt payments (42 CFR 413.89(i)). Because the portion of cost sharing that is not paid by a state's crossover policy counts as bad debt, Medicare's bad debt policy has financial implications for providers serving individuals dually enrolled in Medicare and Medicaid.

For Medicare beneficiaries not enrolled in Medicaid, providers must make a reasonable effort to collect cost-sharing amounts before claiming them as bad debt. When an individual is also enrolled in Medicaid, however, providers are prohibited from attempting to collect Medicare's deductible or coinsurance from the enrollee. Thus, if a state does not cover Medicare's full cost sharing, the uncovered amount may be reimbursed as bad debt. As a result, providers may be able

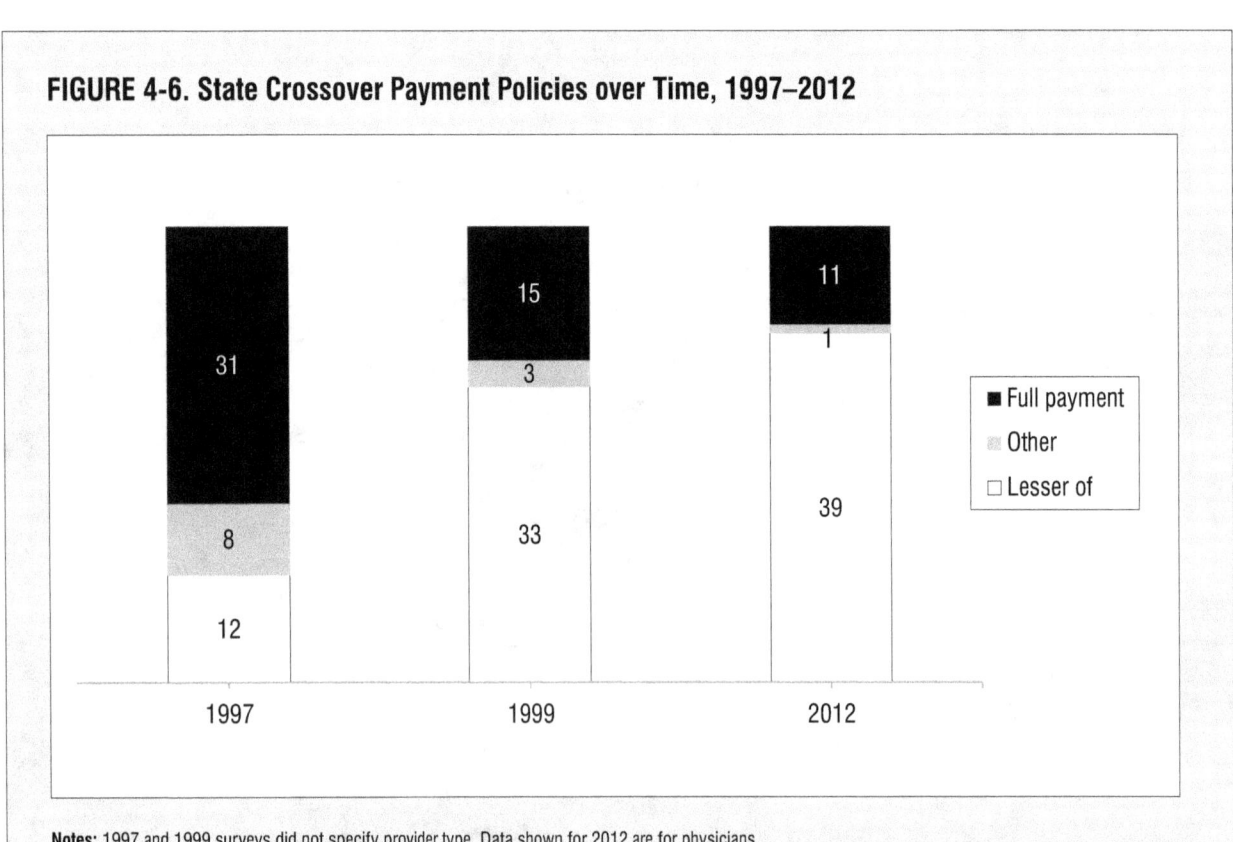

FIGURE 4-6. State Crossover Payment Policies over Time, 1997–2012

Notes: 1997 and 1999 surveys did not specify provider type. Data shown for 2012 are for physicians.
Sources: 1997 and 1999 data are taken from surveys of State Medicaid Directors conducted by the National Senior Citizens Law Center and the Kaiser Family Foundation (Nemore 1999); 2012 data were collected by NORC at the University of Chicago for MACPAC.

to recoup from Medicare a portion of the cost sharing that Medicaid programs do not pay.

Unpaid cost sharing from crossover claims may account for a substantial portion of bad debt. Nationwide, the American Hospital Association estimates that individuals dually enrolled in Medicaid and Medicare account for 20 percent of Medicare beneficiaries, but 55 percent of hospitals' Medicare bad debt (AHA 2011). The American Health Care Association estimates that dual eligibles account for nearly 94 percent of unpaid SNF copayments (AHCA 2012).

It appears that some states have considered providers' ability to recoup unpaid cost-sharing amounts through bad debt when deciding whether to implement lesser-of policies, and some make explicit mention of the availability of bad debt reimbursement from Medicare in explaining their policy. For example, Oklahoma's announcement of a change from a full-copay policy to a lesser-of policy for hospitals suggested that hospitals should look into Medicare's bad debt criteria (OHCA 2010).

Data limitations regarding Medicaid payment of Medicare coinsurance and deductibles

The total amount of Medicare cost sharing paid by the Medicaid program cannot be readily discerned from federal data sources. In some cases, cost-sharing amounts are reported on the Form CMS-64 expenditure report separately from other services, and in others it appears that cost-sharing payments are reported as payments for the underlying service (e.g., inpatient hospital, nursing facility). This may be particularly true in the case of cost sharing for non-QMB full-benefit dual eligibles. Instructions for the CMS-64 indicate that separate reporting is intended to capture cost-sharing amounts only for QMBs, but this may not be done consistently. There may also be cases where claims do not cross over automatically from the Medicare program, and providers must submit claims for cost-sharing amounts directly to the Medicaid program. In these cases, the claims may not always be reflected in federal claims data such as the Medicaid Statistical Information System.

Policy Implications

These findings raise several important issues regarding the interaction of Medicaid and Medicare payment policies, as well as the potential effects of these policies on enrollees' access to services. For one, Medicaid coverage of Medicare deductibles and coinsurance and Medicare bad debt payment result in shifting costs between the programs. For example, if states reduce their payment rates for hospitals and nursing facilities, Medicare bad debt payments increase. Conversely, if the Medicare program increases coinsurance requirements, then Medicaid spending, shared by the states and federal government, increases. Interactions are further complicated when dual eligibles are enrolled in Medicaid managed care plans or Medicare Advantage plans, in which case claims may not automatically cross over to the responsible payer.

The Medicare Payment Advisory Commission has previously raised these interactions and resultant cost shifting as issues (MedPAC 2004). At the same time, administrative resources to enroll individuals in MSP programs and process claims for premiums, deductibles, and coinsurance are also affected by state and federal coverage and payment policies.

The impact of state payment policies for Medicare cost sharing on beneficiary access to services is unclear. Both providers and beneficiary advocates contend that state Medicaid policies to limit payment of Medicare cost sharing leads to insufficient access to needed services for dual eligibles. The ability of certain providers to recoup a portion of unpaid cost sharing through Medicare bad debt payment may mitigate the potential negative effects on access that might result from state policies that limit cost-sharing payments. However, physicians are not eligible for bad debt payment, and at least one study found that access to outpatient physician visits for dually eligible beneficiaries was reduced relative to non-dually eligible beneficiaries in states that limited their Medicare cost-sharing payment amounts (Thompson 2003).

While these findings are suggestive, a more complete understanding of the effect of state payment policies for Medicare cost sharing on access to health care services for dual eligibles would require information on the differences between Medicaid and Medicare payment rates in each state, the number of providers that serve dual eligibles, and the use of services among dual eligibles. Further research could also provide insight into the extent to which state policies to limit payment of deductibles and coinsurance affect total payments to providers. Understanding this effect would require additional information regarding the amount of unpaid cost sharing, by state and type of service.

Further, in many cases, state Medicaid payments for Medicare cost sharing will be affected by Medicaid primary care payment requirements in 2013 and 2014. Federal statute requires that, for these two years, Medicaid programs pay primary care physicians for primary care services at rates that are at least equal to Medicare (§1902(a)(13)(C) of the Act). As a result, even in the 41 states that limit their Medicare cost-sharing payments for physicians, primary care providers will receive the full amount of Medicare cost sharing for primary care services in 2013 and 2014.

The Commission will continue to explore the role that states play in assuring access to services for dual eligibles, including state enrollment policies and the effect of state Medicaid payment policies for Medicare cost sharing.

Endnotes

1 Figures are from a Mathematica Policy Research analysis of 2007 Medicare and Medicaid data for MACPAC and MACPAC analysis of CMS-64 Financial Management Report net expenditure data. The total amount of Medicare cost sharing paid by the Medicaid program can be difficult to discern from federal data sources because cost-sharing amounts are sometimes reported separately and other times reported as payments for the underlying service.

2 If the amount paid by Medicare exceeds the Medicaid rate, then these states make no additional payment for coinsurance or deductibles.

3 Medicare Part C (Medicare Advantage) is operated through Medicare-approved private insurance plans, includes all benefits and services covered under Part A and Part B, usually includes Medicare prescription drug coverage (Part D), and may include extra benefits and services. Beneficiaries enrolled in Part C plans are responsible for paying monthly Part B premiums and, depending on their chosen plan, may be responsible for a monthly premium to the Medicare plan, copayments, coinsurance, and deductibles.

4 Although much of the MCCA was repealed in the following year, the QMB program remained in law as section 1902(a)(10)(E) of the Social Security Act. Prior to the MCCA, Congress had enacted the Omnibus Budget and Reconciliation Act of 1986, which gave states the option to either offer Medicaid coverage of Medicare cost sharing or expand full Medicaid benefit coverage to low-income Medicare beneficiaries with incomes up to 100 percent FPL and resources not in excess of the SSI resource level. The option to expand full Medicaid benefits to those with incomes up to 100 percent FPL still exists, and currently, 22 states and the District of Columbia use this option (see MACStats Table 11).

5 Medicaid also pays the Part A premiums for a small number of QMBs. These are individuals who are required to pay Part A premiums because they do not have sufficient work history to quality for Social Security.

6 The QI program was most recently extended via the American Taxpayer Relief Act of 2012 (P.L. 112-240, §621) through December 2013.

7 States do not receive FFP for Part B premiums for non-MSP dual eligibles if the state elects this option (42 CFR §431.625(d)(1); see OIG 2012d). States also cannot receive FFP for covering services that could have been paid for by Medicare Part B if the eligible recipient had been enrolled in Medicare (§1903(b)(1)).

8 These estimates do not include individuals who are also eligible for full Medicaid benefits. Enrollment rates for full-benefit dual eligibles are estimated to be higher.

9 States may require QMBs to pay a small amount of cost sharing, consistent with the amounts paid by other (non-dual) Medicaid enrollees.

10 Medicaid enrollees in an institution, and certain enrollees receiving home and community-based waiver services, may be required to contribute a portion of any income to the cost of their Medicaid services. Their contribution is determined by subtracting from their income a personal needs allowance and allowances for a spouse or other dependents living in the community. Regulations regarding post-eligibility treatment of income can be found at 42 CFR 435.725–735, 435.832, and 436.832.

11 If states contract with managed care plans to cover their Medicare cost-sharing obligations, the capitation rate must take into account the payment levels specified in the Medicaid state plan and the methodology for determining the capitation rate must be part of the approved Medicaid state plan.

12 Bad debt is paid under fee-for-service Medicare only. CMS does not pay providers for the unpaid cost sharing of Medicare managed care plan members.

References

American Health Care Association (AHCA). 2012. Bad debt "lifeline" must be protected. Washington, DC: AHCA. http://www.ahcancal.org/News/publication/AHCA_Notes/AHCA%20Notes,%20February%202012.pdf.

American Hospital Association (AHA). 2011. Assistance to low-income Medicare beneficiaries (bad debt). Washington, DC: AHA. http://www.aha.org/content/12/fs-bad-debt.pdf.

Carpenter, L. 1998. Evolution of Medicaid coverage of Medicare cost sharing. *Health Care Financing Review* 20, no. 2: 11–18. https://www.cms.gov/Research-Statistics-Data-and-Systems/Research/HealthCareFinancingReview/downloads/98winterpg11.pdf.

Centers for Medicare & Medicaid Services (CMS), U.S. Department of Health and Human Services. 2013a. *Data Analysis Brief: Medicare-Medicaid Dual Enrollment from 2006 through 2011*. Baltimore, MD: CMS. http://www.cms.gov/Medicare-Medicaid-Coordination/Medicare-and-Medicaid-Coordination/Medicare-Medicaid-Coordination-Office/Downloads/Dual_Enrollment_2006-2011_Final_Document.pdf.

Centers for Medicare & Medicaid Services (CMS), U.S. Department of Health and Human Services. 2013b. Medicare costs at a glance. Baltimore, MD: CMS. http://www.medicare.gov/your-medicare-costs/costs-at-a-glance/costs-at-glance.html.

Centers for Medicare & Medicaid Services (CMS), U.S. Department of Health and Human Services. 2012a. Dual eligibles and Medicare cost sharing. Baltimore, MD: CMS. http://www.medicaid.gov/State-Resource-Center/Frequently-Asked-Questions/Downloads/Medicare-Cost-Sharing-FAQ.pdf.

Centers for Medicare & Medicaid Services (CMS), U.S. Department of Health and Human Services. 2012b. *Medicaid coverage of Medicare beneficiaries (dual eligibles) at a glance*. Baltimore, MD: CMS. http://www.cms.gov/Outreach-and-Education/Medicare-Learning-Network-MLN/MLNProducts/downloads/Medicare_Beneficiaries_Dual_Eligibles_At_a_Glance.pdf.

Centers for Medicare & Medicaid Services (CMS), U.S. Department of Health and Human Services. 2006. Medicare program: Revisions to payment policies, five-year review of work relative value units, changes to the practice expense methodology under the physician fee schedule, and other changes to payment under Part B. Final rule. *Federal Register* 71, no. 231 (December 1): 69624–70251.

Committee on the Budget, U.S. House of Representatives. 1990. *Report of the Committee on the Budget, House of Representatives to Accompany H.R. 5835*. House Report 101-964.

Congressional Budget Office (CBO). 2004. *A description of CBO's cost estimate for the Medicare prescription drug benefit*. Washington, DC: CBO. http://www.cbo.gov/sites/default/files/cbofiles/ftpdocs/56xx/doc5668/07-21-medicare.pdf.

Glaun, K. 2002. *Medicaid programs to assist low-income Medicare beneficiaries: Medicare savings programs case studies*. Washington, DC: Kaiser Commission on Medicaid and the Uninsured. http://www.kff.org/medicaid/upload/Medicaid-Programs-to-Assist-Low-Income-Medicare-Beneficiaries-Medicare-Savings-Programs-Case-Study-Findings-Background-Paper.pdf.

Haber, S.G., W. Adamache, E. Walsh, et al. 2003. *Evaluation of qualified Medicare beneficiary (QMB) and specified low-income Medicare beneficiary (SLMB) programs*. Final report, Volume 1. Waltham, MA: RTI International. Report to CMS, CMS contract no. 500-95-5008. http://www.cms.gov/Research-Statistics-Data-and-Systems/Statistics-Trends-and-Reports/Reports/downloads/HaberVol1.pdf.

Health Care Financing Administration (HCFA), U.S. Department of Health and Human Services. 1997. Letter from Sally K. Richardson to State Medicaid Directors regarding "Section 4714 of the Balanced Budget Act." November 24, 1997. http://downloads.cms.gov/cmsgov/archived-downloads/SMDL/downloads/SMD112497.pdf.

Health Care Financing Administration (HCFA), U.S. Department of Health and Human Services. 1991. Chapter 3. In *State Medicaid Manual*. Baltimore, MD: HCFA. https://www.cms.gov/Regulations-and-Guidance/Guidance/Manuals/Paper-Based-Manuals-Items/CMS021927.html.

Medicare Payment Advisory Commission (MedPAC). 2004. Chapter 3. Dual eligible beneficiaries: An overview. In *Report to the Congress: New approaches in Medicare*. June 2004. Washington, DC: MedPAC. http://www.medpac.gov/publications/congressional_reports/June04_ch3.pdf.

Nemore, P. 1999. *Variations in state Medicaid buy-in practices for low-income Medicare beneficiaries: A 1999 update*. Washington, DC: Henry J. Kaiser Family Foundation. http://www.kff.org/medicaid/1566-index.cfm.

Nemore, P., J.A. Bender, and W. Kwok 2006. *Toward making Medicare work for low-income beneficiaries: A baseline comparison of the Part D low-income subsidy and Medicare savings programs eligibility and enrollment rules*. Washington, DC: Henry J. Kaiser Family Foundation. http://www.kff.org/medicare/7519.cfm.

Neumann, P.J., M.D. Bernardin, E.J. Bayer, et al. 1994. *Identifying barriers to elderly participation in the qualified Medicare beneficiary program*. Prepared for the Health Care Financing Administration under Cooperative Agreement No. 17-C-90094/3-01. Bethesda, MD: Project Hope Center for Health Affairs.

Nonnemaker, L., and S. Sinclair. 2011. *Medicare beneficiaries' out-of-pocket spending for health care*. Washington, DC: AARP Public Policy Institute. http://assets.aarp.org/rgcenter/ppi/health-care/i48-oop.pdf.

Office of Inspector General (OIG), U.S. Department of Health and Human Services. 2012a. *Arizona improperly claimed federal reimbursement for Medicare Part B premiums paid on behalf of Medicaid beneficiaries*. Report no. A-09-11-02009. Washington, DC: OIG. https://oig.hhs.gov/oas/reports/region9/91102009.pdf.

Office of Inspector General (OIG), U.S. Department of Health and Human Services. 2012b. *Montana did not properly pay Medicare Part B deductibles and coinsurance for outpatient services*. Report no. A-07-11-03172. Washington, DC: OIG. http://oig.hhs.gov/oas/reports/region7/71103172.pdf.

Office of Inspector General (OIG), U.S. Department of Health and Human Services. 2012c. *Nebraska did not properly pay some Medicare Part B deductibles and coinsurance*. Report no. A-07-11-03168. Washington, DC: OIG. http://oig.hhs.gov/oas/reports/region7/71103168.pdf.

Office of Inspector General (OIG), U.S. Department of Health and Human Services. 2012d. *Review of Nebraska's Medicaid payments for dual eligible individuals' Medicare Part A deductibles and coinsurance*. Report no. A-07-11-03161. Washington, DC: OIG. http://oig.hhs.gov/oas/reports/region7/71103161.asp.

Oklahoma Health Care Authority (OHCA). 2010. *SoonerCare reimbursement notice: Hospital updates*. OHCA PRN 2010-03, March 11, 2010. Oklahoma City, OK: OHCA. http://www.okhca.org/WorkArea/linkit.aspx?LinkIdentifier=id&ItemID=11536.

Rosenbach, M., and J. Lamphere. 1999. *Bridging the gaps between Medicare and Medicaid: The case of QMBs and SLMBs*. Washington, DC: AARP. http://assets.aarp.org/rgcenter/health/9902_qmbs.pdf.

Social Security Administration (SSA). 2012. Resource limits for subsidy eligibility. Baltimore, MD: SSA. https://secure.ssa.gov/apps10/poms.nsf/lnx/0603030025.

Summer, L. 2006. *Accomplishments and lessons from the State Solutions initiative to increase enrollment in the Medicare savings programs*. New Brunswick, NJ: Rutgers Center for State Health Policy. https://gushare.georgetown.edu/xythoswfs/webui/_xy-6486017_2-t_lJWtqz3E.

Summer, L., and R. Friedland. 2002. *The role of the asset test in targeting benefits for Medicare savings programs*. Washington, DC: The Commonwealth Fund. http://www.commonwealthfund.org/publications/publications_show.htm?doc_id=221324.

Thompson, T. 2003. *Report to the Congress on state payment limitations for Medicare cost sharing*. Washington, DC: U.S. Department of Health and Human Services.

U.S. Government Accountability Office (GAO). 2012. *Medicare savings programs: Implementation of requirements aimed at increasing enrollment*. Washington, DC: GAO. Report GAO_12-871. http://www.gao.gov/assets/650/648370.pdf.

Waxman, S.P., F.W. Hunger, B.C. Biddle, et al. 1997. Brief for the federal respondent in opposition in California Ambulance Association, et al., v. Shalala, et al. (no. 97-1949); and Gilmore, et al., v. Shalala, et al. (no. 97-2079) and brief for the United States as amicus curiae supporting respondent in Beverly Community Hospital Association, et al. v. Belshé (no. 97-1947). Ninth Circuit Court of Appeals. http://www.justice.gov/osg/briefs/1997/0responses/97-1947.resp.pdf.

CHAPTER 5

Issues in Setting Medicaid Capitation Rates for Integrated Care Plans

Key Points

Issues in Setting Medicaid Capitation Rates for Integrated Care Plans

- Many states serve persons dually eligible for Medicare and Medicaid through risk-based managed care plans that integrate Medicare and Medicaid services, and several more states have proposed new capitated models under the Centers for Medicare & Medicaid Services (CMS) financial alignment demonstrations. How CMS and the states approach setting Medicaid capitation rates for plans participating in these programs will be a key factor in determining whether these programs move forward, can be sustained over time, and meet expectations for financial savings.

- Challenges for states in setting Medicaid capitation payment rates for integrated care plans include accounting for the wide variability in enrollee use of long-term services and supports (LTSS) and balancing financial incentives with acceptable plan risk. Ideally, the capitation rates should be set at levels that are neither so low that plans avoid enrolling individuals with the greatest needs or limit access to services, nor so high that there are no incentives for plans to be efficient.

- States have experience with two existing integrated care programs for dual eligibles: (1) state arrangements with Medicare Advantage dual-eligible special needs plans (D-SNPs) and (2) Program of All-inclusive Care for the Elderly (PACE) plans. These states use a range of rate-setting tools to create financial incentives while accounting for population differences and financial risk to the plans.

- Voluntary enrollment can make rate setting more challenging because the average health and functional status of the population that ultimately enrolls in the program may be significantly different from the population characteristics assumed in the rate-setting process. Rate-setting mechanisms that adjust for population differences can help account for voluntary enrollment.

- Only a few states have implemented a Medicaid risk adjustment process for dual eligibles because the commonly used risk adjustment models are limited in their ability to predict LTSS costs. Risk adjustment models that are more predictive of Medicaid LTSS costs will likely be needed as more states serve dual eligibles through risk-based managed care programs. Given the differences in LTSS benefits in each state, a single risk adjustment model may not accurately predict LTSS costs across states, and some states may need to develop their own models.

CHAPTER 5

Issues in Setting Medicaid Capitation Rates for Integrated Care Plans

Individuals over age 65 and younger persons with disabilities who are dually eligible for both Medicare and Medicaid (dual eligibles) are among the highest-need and highest-cost individuals in both programs. As a result, they have become the focus of efforts to develop more effective integrated care delivery models. The goal of these programs is to provide better coordination of Medicare and Medicaid services, lower costs, and improve health and functional outcomes for this population.

Several states are serving dual eligibles through risk-based managed care models, and more have proposed to do so. Under these models, the state pays participating managed care plans a capitated payment—a fixed amount for a defined package of benefits, usually paid on a per member per month basis. The managed care plan assumes financial risk for the cost of covered services and plan administration. The combination of a fixed payment amount and financial risk is intended to create incentives for the managed care plan to coordinate care so that needed services are provided in the most cost-effective manner.

Among the states that have moved to capitated managed care for dual eligibles, some have created arrangements with Medicare Advantage dual-eligible special needs plans (D-SNPs) and developed Program of All-inclusive Care for the Elderly (PACE) programs to coordinate Medicaid and Medicare benefits. The Centers for Medicare & Medicaid Services (CMS) is working with states on initiatives to create new integrated care plan options and further coordinate services for dual eligibles.

The largest initiatives in this effort are the financial alignment demonstrations, in which 15 states are working with CMS to enroll dual eligibles into risk-based managed care.[1] Estimates are that up to 2 million individuals could be enrolled in the financial alignment demonstrations in the future (Bella 2012). Under these managed care models, CMS and the states will collaborate to develop care delivery approaches that encourage more coordination across Medicare and Medicaid services. Both Medicare and Medicaid will share in the savings achieved through the demonstrations.

Much of the public attention to the financial alignment demonstrations has focused on how care management, enrollment, and appeals processes will be approached, and how savings resulting from the demonstrations will be allocated and used. Another important issue is how the capitation rates will be set. The approach to setting capitation rates for plans participating in these programs will be a key factor in determining whether the demonstrations move forward, are sustained over time, and meet expectations for financial savings.

This chapter focuses on several policy and technical issues related to setting appropriate Medicaid capitation rates for integrated care programs serving dual eligibles. It begins with an overview of the general Medicaid capitation rate-setting process for dual eligibles and highlights the significance of enrollees' use of long-term services and supports (LTSS) in developing these rates. The chapter then describes various components of rate-setting methodologies that states have used to develop capitation rates in existing integrated dual-eligible managed care programs and provides state-specific examples of the joint rate-setting process being used for CMS's financial alignment demonstrations. The chapter concludes by raising additional policy issues for consideration.

Overview of Rate Setting for Medicaid Managed Care

Today, several states have plans that serve dual eligibles through Medicaid capitated arrangements. Many of these plans also participate in the Medicare Advantage program and receive capitated payments from CMS to provide Medicare benefits for beneficiaries who have chosen to enroll. Typically, when a beneficiary is enrolled in the same plan for both Medicare and Medicaid, the plan receives separately developed Medicare and Medicaid capitation rates.

Medicaid capitation rate-setting methods vary from state to state. This section describes some of the key concepts in developing capitation rates for Medicaid enrollees and some of the challenges in setting rates for dual eligibles. Later sections address how states have implemented these concepts in developing capitation rates for integrated care models, such as D-SNPs, PACE, and the financial alignment demonstrations.

Medicare capitation rates for D-SNP and PACE plans are developed as part of the national Medicare Advantage and Part D rate-setting and bid processes and are not discussed in this chapter.[2]

Capitation rate development

In determining Medicaid capitation rates, states begin with a baseline of historical claims and eligibility data for the relevant population and make adjustments to reflect expected costs during the payment period (typically one year). Using the adjusted baseline, capitation rates are set for groups of enrollees to reflect differences in predicted service use for each group. States may further refine their payment methodologies with various approaches to mitigate some of the plans' financial risk and to create incentives related to plan performance and quality of care. Ideally, the capitation rates should be set at levels that are neither so low that plans avoid enrolling individuals with the greatest needs or limit access to services, nor so high that there are no incentives for plans to be efficient.

Establishing and adjusting the baseline. The rate-setting process starts by establishing a baseline of historical spending for the relevant population. The baseline data are typically one to two years of recent experience for the eligible population and are based on either fee-for-service (FFS) claims or managed care plan encounter data. The services included in the baseline data reflect those included in the managed care contract; any services carved out of the contract would be excluded from the baseline.

The baseline data are then adjusted for several factors, including:

- claims completion (i.e., services provided for which a claim has not yet been paid);
- state or federal policy and programmatic changes (e.g., fee schedule and benefit package changes);
- price and utilization trends;
- anticipated managed care efficiency (e.g., if the baseline uses FFS data, expected differences in service price and utilization realized through managed care); and
- administrative costs (including care management activities not routinely conducted under FFS).

Determining rate cells. Rather than paying the same rate for every enrollee, states develop Medicaid capitation rates for subgroups of the enrolled population who have similar cost characteristics. These subpopulation-specific rates are called rate cells. The rate cells may be based on enrollee characteristics such as basis of eligibility, age, gender, and geographic region.

Risk adjustment. Risk adjustment may be used in Medicaid managed care programs to further refine payments to plans based on enrollee health status and service needs. Risk adjustment approaches typically use diagnostic information and other enrollee characteristics to calculate a risk score that represents an individual enrollee's expected costs relative to the average cost of the overall population.

The risk score is applied to the capitation rate so that a plan is paid more for enrollees with higher-acuity conditions and less for enrollees with lower-acuity conditions. Risk adjustment can protect against unintended incentives for adverse selection or "cherry picking" healthier enrollees among health plans. The use of rate cells and risk adjustment allows for payment to vary based on enrollee characteristics when there is a different enrollment mix across participating plans.

Risk sharing. States may use risk-sharing arrangements such as risk corridors or stop-loss provisions to mitigate some of the plan's financial risk. Under risk corridors, the state limits a plan's gains and losses by sharing in the costs or savings beyond a certain threshold. The state will reimburse the plan for a certain percentage of losses if aggregate spending for services exceeds the plan's capitation payments and will share in a portion of the savings should payments for services be less than the capitation payments.

Stop-loss or reinsurance provisions protect plans from losses beyond predetermined thresholds on an individual basis (e.g., $100,000 in annual payments for a single enrollee). Beyond the specified threshold, the state will assume some or all of the enrollee's cost of care. If stop-loss or reinsurance provisions are used to limit the amount of loss a plan may experience, the capitation rates are adjusted to account for the reduced risk that the plans bear.

Incentive and withhold payments. States may include incentive payments in the rate-setting process that give plans a bonus for achieving high ratings on performance or quality measures. Alternatively, the state may withhold a small percentage of the capitation payment and allow the plan to earn it back by meeting certain performance standards.

Challenges in Medicaid rate setting for dual eligibles

There are several challenges for states in setting capitation payment rates for dual eligibles under Medicaid, including accounting for enrollee use of LTSS and balancing a state's desire for savings with acceptable plan risk.

Accounting for LTSS. Spending on LTSS accounts for approximately 70 percent of Medicaid benefit spending for full-benefit dual eligibles (see Chapter 3 of this report), so a key element of the Medicaid rate-setting process for this population is how the state calculates the portion of the rate that covers LTSS. Theoretically, putting plans at risk for LTSS should create incentives for plans to provide services in the most cost-effective setting, for example, assisting certain individuals in the community, rather than in a nursing facility setting.

Experience with paying plans on a capitated basis for LTSS varies across the states. In the majority of states, LTSS users and services have typically been carved out of the managed care program and claims have been paid on a FFS basis. In 2012, 16 states operated capitated LTSS programs that covered nearly 400,000 LTSS users (Saucier et al. 2012). Additionally, capitated LTSS may be delivered through PACE plans. There were about 25,000 PACE enrollees across 29 states in 2012 (National PACE Association 2012).

Balancing savings and plan risk. Another challenge in developing capitation rates for Medicaid managed care plans for dual eligibles is balancing the desire a state may have for savings through managed care with the financial risk plans face in delivering services for this diverse population. Some dual eligibles are relatively healthy and require very few services, while others have multiple chronic health conditions and functional limitations that require a nursing facility stay or other institutional care. Consequently, the financial risks to plans are considerable should the needs of its enrolled population not match the cost and savings assumptions built into the capitation rates. Yet if states go too far in constraining the risks that plans face, they might also reduce the incentives for plans to seek out cost-effective ways to deliver services.

The wide variability in LTSS use and spending is the key driver of financial risk to the plans. Even among enrollees who have been certified to need a nursing facility level of care, the LTSS needs of frail persons age 65 and over may be very different from the LTSS needs of individuals with physical or intellectual disabilities. The average Medicaid cost per all-year, full-benefit dual-eligible enrollee who does not use any LTSS was about $2,800 in 2007, compared to approximately $32,000 for those who use home and community-based (HCBS) wavier services and approximately $44,000 for enrollees who use institutional LTSS services (see Chapter 3 of this report).

Current Experience with Managed Care for Dual-Eligible Enrollees

For states that enroll dual eligibles in a Medicaid managed care plan, the level of coordination with the Medicare program and with Medicare Advantage plans can vary. While states may make enrollment into a managed care plan mandatory or voluntary for Medicaid benefits, beneficiary enrollment into a Medicare Advantage plan is voluntary.[3] In some states, individuals may be enrolled in separate managed care plans for their Medicare and Medicaid benefits or they may receive their Medicare benefits through FFS while being enrolled in a managed care plan for Medicaid. Other states have made a push to voluntarily enroll dual eligibles in one plan for both programs, to create an integrated care program.

States' experiences with Medicare Advantage D-SNP and PACE plans shed light on some of the key design issues in setting capitation rates for integrated care plans serving dual eligibles. This section provides an overview of the Medicaid rate-setting processes for these plans. Key rate-setting design issues are highlighted, particularly regarding how states determine the right balance between nursing facility services and HCBS in setting the capitation rates and the use of risk mitigation strategies. In the following section, we touch upon rate setting under the financial alignment demonstrations that are expected to begin soon in a few states.

State arrangements with dual-eligible special needs plans

Many Medicaid managed care plans serving dual eligibles participate in the Medicare Advantage program as D-SNPs—Medicare Advantage plans designed to provide targeted care to individuals dually eligible for Medicare and Medicaid. State Medicaid contracts with D-SNPs vary in the types of Medicaid services covered, with some states carving out one or more services, such as behavioral health or nursing facility services, from the contract.

Fully integrated dual-eligible (FIDE) SNPs. D-SNPs that have risk-based contracts with state Medicaid agencies to provide specified acute care services, LTSS, and coordination of Medicare and Medicaid services are considered to be fully integrated plans (42 CFR 422.2). Five states require Medicaid managed care plans serving dual eligibles to be FIDE SNPs, and require enrollees that wish to voluntarily enroll in the integrated program to choose the same managed care entity for both sets of benefits (Saucier et al. 2012). Only a small number of Medicare Advantage D-SNP plans have contracted with states to become FIDE SNPs. In 2008, an estimated 120,000 dual eligibles were enrolled in D-SNPs that also had Medicaid contracts (Bella and Palmer 2009).

For Medicaid, there are no requirements regarding the categories of dual eligibles that may enroll in a FIDE SNP. States may choose to include only a certain subset of dual eligibles in a FIDE SNP plan, such as those who receive full Medicaid benefits or those who meet nursing facility level of care criteria.

Capitation payments. Medicaid capitation payments to FIDE SNPs must comply with the same statutory requirement for actuarial soundness that applies to other Medicaid managed care programs (MACPAC 2011).[4] States have used a variety of rate-setting design options to create incentives for providing LTSS in the most cost-effective setting while mitigating some of the risk to the plans in providing these services.

Use of rate cells. For FIDE SNP plans, typical Medicaid capitation rate cells might include age (under 65 and over 65 years), geography, and frailty level or institutional status. Creating separate rate cells based on institutional status may help mitigate risk for the plan, but it does not create strong incentives to maintain an individual in the community as the plan will get a payment increase once the enrollee is institutionalized. If states use separate rates for institutional status, they may include other payment structures to create stronger incentives to keep the enrollee in the community.

For example, the Massachusetts Senior Care Options (SCO) program utilizes separate rate cells for institutional versus community enrollees, but includes a transition policy to create incentives to maintain an individual in a community setting. For the first three months after an enrollee switches from the community to an institutional setting, or vice versa, the plan will be paid according to the prior level of care. Thus, for a person transitioning from the community to an institutional setting, the plan is paid at the community capitation rate for the first three months. Likewise, for a person transitioning from an institutional setting to the community, the plan is paid at the higher institutional capitation rate for three months (Massachusetts DHHS 2010).

Partial risk arrangements for LTSS. Because LTSS can be so expensive, some states limit the amount of risk that plans must take on in this area. These states typically put plans at full risk for HCBS but lessen the amount of risk plans have for nursing facility services. Alternatively, they may create a separate add-on component for nursing facility care. For example, Texas has carved out nursing facility services from its STAR+PLUS program, while the Minnesota Senior Health Options (MSHO) program has put plans at limited risk for nursing facility services.

States sometimes pair limited risk arrangements with other design features to provide an incentive to keep enrollees in the community. For example, Texas withholds 5 percent of the premium from STAR+PLUS plans, which the managed care organizations can earn back if they meet performance standards on several measures, including no statistically significant increase in the nursing facility admission rate (Texas HHSC 2012).

In Minnesota, MSHO plans are at risk only for the first 180 days of nursing facility care. The plans are paid a separate add-on payment intended to cover potential nursing facility placements, which is paid to the plan for all enrollees living in the community. Once a person is admitted to a nursing facility, the add-on payment is stopped and the plan covers up to 180 days of nursing facility care out of the previously paid add-on revenues (Minnesota DHS 2012).

Risk sharing. States may use risk-sharing arrangements such as risk corridors to limit a plan's gains and losses by sharing in the costs or savings beyond a certain threshold. For example, the Massachusetts SCO program established four risk corridors for the first few years of the program.[5] For gains or losses between 0 and 5 percent of the plan's capitation revenue, the plan bore all of the losses or kept all of the gains. Massachusetts was responsible for 50 percent of the losses or kept 50 percent of the gains between 5 and 15 percent of the plan's capitation revenue, and 75 percent of losses or gains between 15 and 25 percent of revenue. The plan bore all of the losses or kept all of the gains greater than 25 percent.

Some states have created specialized risk-sharing arrangements around a specific benefit or assumptions used in the rate-setting process. In Arizona's Long Term Care System program, the LTSS portion of the capitation rate is based in part on an assumed ratio of HCBS and nursing facility months for each plan. If a plan's HCBS nursing facility mix is 1 percent over or under this assumed mix percentage, the plan bears all of the costs or retains all of the savings. If the difference is greater than 1 percent over or under the assumed mix, the state and plan share the costs or savings equally (AHCCCS 2012).

Risk adjustment. Risk adjustment is commonly used for high-cost populations in Medicaid managed care to account for differences in the enrollment mix between plans. However, few states have implemented risk adjustment for the Medicaid benefits covered by FIDE SNPs due to the limitations of existing risk adjustment models for LTSS costs. The commonly used risk adjustment models have been designed to predict the cost of acute care services. These models are based largely on demographic factors (e.g., age and sex), health status, and diagnostic information, and their predictive capabilities do not correlate well with LTSS costs.

This limitation of existing risk adjustment models is problematic for determining appropriate

Medicaid payments to FIDE SNP plans, because the most significant risk for plans is for LTSS. In order to have meaningful risk adjustment for the Medicaid capitation rate, the state must implement a risk adjustment model that takes into account functional status and other enrollee characteristics that are more predictive of LTSS needs, such as measures of level of care, activities of daily living (ADLs), and cognition. However, developing and implementing an LTSS risk adjustment process can be resource intensive. If a state is not collecting the same measures of frailty as other states, it may not be able to leverage an existing model and would need to develop its own model to predict LTSS costs. The level of effort required to develop and implement an LTSS risk adjustment process has been a factor in states not putting LTSS services fully at risk in their capitated arrangements with FIDE SNP programs.

One state that has developed an LTSS risk adjustment model is Wisconsin. In the Wisconsin Family Care Partnership program, the state currently puts plans at full risk for nursing facility services and uses risk adjustment to account for a plan's relative risk based on the characteristics of the enrolled population. The state separately risk adjusts the acute care and LTSS components of the Medicaid capitation rate.

For the acute care component of the Medicaid capitation rates, Wisconsin uses the hierarchical condition category (HCC) model used by Medicare to risk adjust plan payments for Medicare Advantage plans. For the LTSS component of the Medicaid capitation rate, a separate regression model takes into account the enrollee's functional status as well as certain health-related conditions. In addition, the state has developed three separate LTSS regression models for persons with developmental disabilities, persons with physical disabilities, and persons age 65 and over because the average costs and the most predictive measures are different for each of these populations (Wisconsin DHS 2012).

Program of All-Inclusive Care for the Elderly

PACE provides another integrated service delivery model that involves risk-based capitated payments from both Medicare and Medicaid. PACE is a covered Medicare service and is available as a Medicaid service as a state plan option. It provides comprehensive medical care, behavioral health services, and LTSS to individuals age 55 and older who meet the state's nursing facility level of care criteria. PACE programs generally enroll dual eligibles; however, Medicare or Medicaid eligibility is not required.[6] Enrollment into a PACE plan is voluntary. There were about 25,000 PACE enrollees across 29 states in 2012 (National PACE Association 2012).

Upper payment limit and capitation payments. PACE Medicaid capitation rates are subject to different regulations and guidelines than those that govern rate setting for other Medicaid managed care programs. They are not subject to the actuarial soundness requirement but are instead subject to an upper payment limit (UPL).[7] The UPL is defined as the amount that would otherwise have been paid under the state plan if the participants had not been enrolled in the PACE program (42 CFR 460.182). Even though not required to do so, many states have actuaries set the PACE UPL and capitation rates and follow similar principles and methodologies that would be used to set actuarially sound rates.

The process for determining the UPL is similar to the process used for setting the baseline for other Medicaid capitation rates: historical experience for the PACE-eligible population is adjusted for claims completion and policy and programmatic changes, and then trended forward to the payment period to estimate what expected costs would be for the population if not enrolled in PACE. Most states calculate the UPL first and then set the capitation rate as a fixed percentage of the UPL (e.g., 95 percent of the UPL). This is similar to the adjustment states make to account for the efficiency of managed care compared to a FFS-based baseline. Administrative costs are also included in the PACE capitation rates.

PACE UPL and capitation rates must be based on the costs of comparable populations similar in health and functional status to PACE enrollees. Because most dual eligibles and LTSS services are not covered under managed care programs, the UPL is typically based on the FFS experience of the nursing facility-certifiable population that is using either HCBS waiver or nursing facility services. Unlike many state arrangements with D-SNPs, PACE plans are required to cover all Medicaid state plan approved services, so no services are carved out of the capitation rate and the plans are at full risk for LTSS, including the nursing facility benefit.

Rate cells. Federal statute and regulations require Medicaid PACE capitation rates to be a fixed amount regardless of changes in the enrollee's health status during the contract period. Under this requirement, CMS has prohibited states from developing different capitation rates depending on the site of care. As a result, states cannot use separate institutional and community rate cells as found in some Medicaid payments to D-SNPs, and they have fewer options in the capitation rate structure. PACE capitation rates generally use only a few rate cells, with eligibility (Medicaid only versus dual eligible), geography, and age being the primary rate cell determinants.

Frailty adjustment in PACE. Federal statute and regulations also require that PACE Medicaid capitation rates take into account the comparative frailty of PACE enrollees. Most states use the average cost of enrollees using HCBS and nursing facility services as a proxy for frailty (National PACE Association 2009). States typically create a blended capitation rate based on the existing proportion of Medicaid FFS enrollees who use HCBS waiver and nursing facility services, using the average costs for each group. States may adjust the weighting between the two populations to meet their expectations of the PACE plan's ability to maintain persons in the community or to adjust for the increasing frailty of a plan's enrollees over time. Because the HCBS population is typically less costly than the nursing facility population, this weighting between HCBS waiver enrollees and nursing facility enrollees is typically the key driver in determining the overall level of payment and whether the payment is sufficient to cover the risk of the enrolled population.

Risk adjustment and risk sharing in PACE. PACE plans can face significant risk in the capitation rates because the plans are at full risk for the nursing facility benefit and separate rate cells cannot be used for enrollees in institutions and those living in the community. As mentioned above, the weighting between the nursing facility and the HCBS populations used in the blended capitation rate is the main way states adjust for the frailty of the population. As PACE is voluntary, a state may over- or underpay plans if the population that actually enrolls in the PACE program does not reflect the assumptions used to set the rates. States do not have the flexibility to use partial risk arrangements, nursing facility add-ons, or other rate-setting design options to help mitigate this risk.

Few states use risk adjustment in PACE due to the same difficulties they face in risk adjusting rates for D-SNPs. Wisconsin and New York risk adjust for LTSS services in PACE by combining the PACE and D-SNP rate-setting efforts and using the LTSS risk adjustment process for both programs.

Medicaid Payment in the Financial Alignment Demonstrations

The CMS financial alignment demonstrations are testing the concept of coordinating the rate-setting processes between Medicaid and Medicare. Currently, while FIDE SNPs and PACE plans receive payments from both Medicare and Medicaid, the financing is still not fully coordinated: the capitation rates for each program are developed independently without full consideration of how a fully integrated, coordinated care program may impact the overall cost of care under the plan. For example, an increase in LTSS services could lead to a decrease in spending on acute care services and overall cost savings; however, states have been reluctant to make this investment as the costs of LTSS are incurred by Medicaid while the initial savings for acute care accrue primarily to Medicare. The financial alignment demonstrations under CMS seek to coordinate the Medicare and Medicaid rate-setting processes to take into account these cross-program interactions and share overall cost savings across both programs.

Joint rate-setting process

CMS has released general guidelines as to how the capitation rates will be set for the financial alignment demonstrations. CMS will make two separate payments, one reflecting coverage of Medicare Part A and B (Medicare A/B) services and one reflecting coverage of Part D services, to the participating health plans for Medicare benefits.[8] The Medicare rate-setting methodology will be consistent across all participating states and will be based on the existing Medicare Advantage and Medicare Part D rate development processes.

The state will make a separate payment to each participating health plan for the Medicaid component of the rate. States and their actuaries, with review from CMS, will develop the Medicaid payment rates (CMS 2013).

Establishing the baseline. CMS will develop Medicare baseline spending estimates, while the states and their actuaries, with review by CMS, will develop the Medicaid baseline spending estimates (CMS 2013). The estimates project what both programs would have spent in the payment year if the demonstration did not exist; this baseline is similar in concept to the UPL used in PACE programs.

The Medicare A/B baseline will be established on a year-by-year basis for each demonstration county. The baseline will be calculated as a weighted average of FFS and Medicare Advantage spending based on the expected proportion of enrollment of beneficiaries who would have previously been in FFS and Medicare Advantage. FFS baseline spending will be based on the published Medicare standardized FFS county rates developed annually as part of the Medicare Advantage rate development process, and the Medicare Advantage spending will reflect the estimated amounts that would have been paid to Medicare Advantage plans in which beneficiaries could enroll. The Part D component will equal the Part D national average monthly bid amount for the payment year (CMS 2013).

The Medicaid baseline will vary by state, based on each state's program design and the historical experience of the target population. The historic spending will use data for the most recent years of prior experience available and will include consideration of Medicaid managed care plan payment (if a state currently serves dual eligibles through capitated managed care) as well as FFS costs (CMS 2013).

Savings targets. An aggregate savings target will be developed and applied to both the Medicaid and

Medicare A/B baseline estimates to determine the capitation payment rates. No savings target will be applied to the Part D component. Medicaid and Medicare will thus share in the savings achieved through the demonstrations.

Based on financial modeling and other analytic work and input from states and others, CMS and the state will establish an aggregate savings target for each year of the demonstration (e.g., 1 percent in year one, 2 percent in year two, and 4 percent in year three). This savings percentage will then be applied prospectively to the Medicare A/B and Medicaid components of the rate. Savings targets may differ among states based on factors such as historic Medicare spending, utilization of institutional LTSS, and penetration of Medicaid managed care. By applying the savings target to the Medicare A/B and Medicaid components, CMS intends to allow both payers to share proportionally in the savings achieved, regardless of whether savings accrue from changes in utilization of acute care services (for which Medicare is the primary payer) or changes in utilization of LTSS services such as nursing facility placements (for which Medicaid is primary) (CMS 2013).

Quality withholds. CMS and the state will withhold a portion of the capitation payments that the participating plans may earn back if they meet certain quality standards. Quality withholds of 1 percent, 2 percent, and 3 percent will be applied to the Medicaid and Medicare A/B components of payment for years one, two, and three respectively; no withhold is applied to the Medicare Part D component (CMS 2013).

Rate cells and risk adjustment. The Medicare A/B and Part D components of the capitation payment will be risk adjusted for the enrollee's health status using the risk adjustment models currently used in Medicare Advantage and Part D (CMS 2013).[9] For Medicaid, states and their actuaries may propose rate cells and risk adjustment for CMS approval, as long as the rate structure creates an incentive for HCBS over institutional placement (CMS 2013). Similar to Medicaid rate setting for FIDE SNPs, Medicaid payment rates under the demonstration may vary at the individual level based on enrollee characteristics such as age, health status, and functional status.

State examples

Massachusetts and Ohio are the first states to have completed memoranda of understanding (MOUs) with CMS for the financial alignment demonstrations that describe the capitation rate structure for the Medicaid component of the rates. Both states have similarities in how the Medicaid capitation rate will be calculated, but each has a unique approach to developing rate cells, implementing risk adjustment, and mitigating financial risk through risk-sharing arrangements (Table 5-1).

Baselines. In Massachusetts and Ohio, the Medicaid baseline spending amounts for each demonstration year will be set up front and will be applied to future years of the demonstration. The baseline estimates will only be revisited to use more recent data or to include an update that results in a substantial change to the baseline (CMS 2012a, CMS 2012b).

Savings targets. The shared savings percentages for Massachusetts and Ohio are set at 1 percent, 2 percent, and 4 percent for years one, two, and three, respectively, and will only be applied to the Medicaid and Medicare A/B components of payment (CMS 2012a, CMS 2012b).

Quality withholds. Both states will apply quality withholds of 1 percent, 2 percent, and 3 percent to the Medicaid and Medicare A/B components of payment for years one, two, and three, respectively (CMS 2012a, CMS 2012b).

Rate cells and risk adjustment. Massachusetts and Ohio have developed different rate structures for rate cells and risk mitigation strategies (CMS 2012a, CMS 2012b). To mitigate risk for the Medicaid component of the rate, Massachusetts will use four rate cells—one facility-based care rate cell for individuals having a long-term facility stay of more than 90 days, and three community rate cells based on LTSS service needs, selected behavioral health conditions, and all other community individuals. Massachusetts will use a high-cost risk pool (HCRP) for select LTSS above a defined threshold within the facility-based and high community needs rate cells to mitigate plan risk and variability across plans for higher than anticipated LTSS costs. The HCRP will be used until an additional LTSS risk adjustment methodology is developed.

In Ohio, the state will segment the population into nursing facility level of care (NFLOC) and "community well" rate cells. Ohio will risk adjust the NFLOC rate cell by using a member enrollment mix adjustment to account for the relative risk and cost differences of major and objectively identifiable subpopulations. This mix adjustment utilizes the particular waiver enrollment and nursing facility placement to provide higher rates to those plans that have a greater proportion of high-risk individuals and lower rates to plans with a lower proportion of high-risk individuals. Additionally, once an enrollee is determined to no longer need NFLOC services, the plan continues to receive the higher NFLOC capitation rate for three months before receiving the lower community well capitation rate in the fourth month.

Risk sharing. Massachusetts will use a risk corridor for the first demonstration year. CMS and Massachusetts only share risk with plans between 5 and 10 percent savings or loss, with a maximum Medicare payment or recoupment equaling 1 percent of the risk-adjusted Medicare baseline and the remaining payments or recoupments treated as Medicaid expenditures eligible for the federal medical assistance percentage. The plans will bear full risk between 0 and 5 percent savings or loss, and for greater than 10 percent savings or loss (CMS 2012a).

In Ohio, CMS and the state will use a minimum medical loss ratio (MMLR) to regulate the minimum amount (as a percentage of the gross joint Medicare and Medicaid payments) that must be used for medical services or expenses related to quality and the care of enrollees. If a plan has a MMLR below 85 percent, the plan must pay back the difference between the 85 percent threshold and the plan's actual MMLR multiplied by the total applicable revenue. The remittance would be distributed back to Medicaid and Medicare based on the proportion each program contributes to the plan's revenue. If the plan's MMLR is between 85 and 90 percent, CMS and the state could require a corrective action plan or levy a fine (CMS 2012b).

Issues for Consideration

States and CMS have shown interest in using integrated care models such as risk-based managed care to provide Medicare and Medicaid services. Through the financial alignment demonstrations, the number of dual eligibles in fully integrated care models could expand greatly: up to 2 million dual eligibles will be eligible to enroll in the demonstration plans. How CMS and the states develop the capitation rates for these plans will be a major factor in determining whether these demonstrations can be successful. Policymakers need to consider several issues when developing the capitation rates, including accounting for voluntary enrollment, the need for LTSS risk

TABLE 5-1. Comparison of Massachusetts and Ohio Medicaid Capitation Rate Elements in Memoranda of Understanding (MOUs) for the Financial Alignment Demonstrations

Rate Element	Massachusetts MOU	Ohio MOU
Baseline costs	Historical state data; trend factors developed by state actuaries with oversight from CMS.	Medicaid capitation rates through the 1915(b) waiver program that would apply for enrollees in the target population but not enrolled in the demo.
Savings percentages	Demo Year 1: 1 percent Demo Year 2: 2 percent Demo Year 3: 4 percent	Demo Year 1: 1 percent Demo Year 2: 2 percent Demo Year 3: 4 percent
Quality withhold	Demo Year 1: 1 percent Demo Year 2: 2 percent Demo Year 3: 3 percent	Demo Year 1: 1 percent Demo Year 2: 2 percent Demo Year 3: 3 percent
Rate cells	Facility-based care: have a long-term facility stay of more than 90 days High community needs: have a skilled need to be met seven days a week; or two or more activities of daily living (ADL) limitations and skilled nursing need three or more days a week; or four or more ADL limitations Community behavioral health: have ongoing, chronic behavioral health condition such as schizophrenia Community other: all other enrollees	Nursing facility level of care (NFLOC): meets a NFLOC as determined through waiver enrollment or 100 or more consecutive days in a nursing facility; single rate cell for each of the seven contracting regions Community well: does not meet a NFLOC standard; three age group (18 to 44, 45 to 64, 65+) rate cells for each of the seven contracting regions Transitional policy: plan receives higher NFLOC rate for three months when enrollee transitions from NFLOC to community well category
Risk adjustment	Rate cells plus a high-cost risk pool (HCRP) for select long-term services and supports spending above a defined threshold. The HCRP will apply to the facility-based care and high community needs rate cells. HCRP will be used until an enhanced risk adjustment methodology is developed.	A member enrollment mix adjustment will be used for the NFLOC rate cell. The relative risk differences of identifiable subpopulations are measured based on particular waiver enrollment and nursing facility placement. Plans with a greater proportion of high-risk individuals get more revenue than plans with lower-risk individuals; adjustments will be budget neutral.

TABLE 5-1, Continued

Rate Element	Massachusetts MOU	Ohio MOU
Risk sharing	Risk corridor established for Demo Year 1. Medicare and Medicaid responsibility is in proportion to contribution to the capitated rate, not including Part D. Maximum Medicare payment or recoupment limited to 1 percent of the risk-adjusted Medicare baseline. Between 0 and 5 percent savings/loss: plans at risk for 100 percent Between 5 and 10 percent savings/loss: plans at risk for 50 percent, CMS and state share other 50 percent (after applying 0 to 5 percent category) Greater than 10 percent savings/loss: plans at risk for 100 percent (after applying other categories)	Each plan must meet Minimum Medical Loss Ratio (MMLR) threshold (as a percentage of the gross combined Medicare and Medicaid payments) beginning in calendar year 2014. If a plan's MMLR is between 85 and 90 percent, state and CMS may require a corrective action plan or levy a fine. Medicaid and Medicare split amount based on each program's percent of revenue to plans. If a plan's MMLR is below 85 percent, the plan must remit the difference between the plan's actual MMLR and the 85 percent threshold multiplied by the total applicable revenue. Medicaid and Medicare split amount based on each program's percent of revenue to plans.

Sources: CMS 2012a, CMS 2012b

adjustment models and appropriate measures of functional status, and the treatment of supplemental payments.

Accounting for voluntary enrollment

A complicating factor in rate setting for dual-eligible managed care programs is the fact that many of these programs have voluntary enrollment, which may lead to an enrolled population that differs in composition from the population experience used in setting the capitation rates. While states are allowed to make enrollment into Medicaid managed care mandatory for dual eligibles, the Medicare program does not allow mandatory enrollment into managed care for Medicare benefits.

Under mandatory managed care enrollment, which is common for other populations in Medicaid, the enrollee characteristics and spending in the baseline experience are likely to be similar to the population that ultimately enrolls, as almost all individuals enroll in the program. Additionally, mandatory-enrollment groups are often large, so that average costs in the past are an actuarially credible predictor of future costs.

In a voluntary program, the average health and functional status of the population that ultimately enrolls in the program may be significantly different from the population used as the baseline experience in the rate-setting process. As a result, there is a chance that the state may over- or underpay, and the plan also faces significant risk of losses. The state must try to adjust the base period experience to account for any differences between the base and the enrolled population. In addition, some programs may only enroll a small number of dual eligibles, making individual enrollees with particularly high costs (i.e., outliers) a significant concern. Effective rate-setting design, such as appropriate rate cells and a good LTSS risk adjustment model, are needed to maintain the positive incentives of risk-based managed care while accurately reflecting the differences in the population enrolled in the program.

Plans participating in the financial alignment demonstrations will all have passive voluntary enrollment, that is, dual eligibles will be automatically enrolled in a managed care plan, but will have the opportunity to voluntarily disenroll from the plan. While other concerns about passive enrollment still remain, from a rate setting perspective, it may increase enrollment and reduce some of the rate-setting issues with voluntary enrollment and small population size. However, some mechanism that adjusts for population differences will still be needed. Additionally, given the uncertainty of the program's costs in the early years, risk mitigation strategies will also be important.

Need for LTSS risk adjustment models

Policymakers seeking to set capitation payments for LTSS struggle to balance the need to create financial incentives for providing services in the most cost-effective setting with the need to ensure plans are paid adequately for a population with significant functional limitations and LTSS needs. Risk adjustment models that are more predictive of Medicaid LTSS costs will likely be needed to help states meet these goals.

Risk adjustment allows the state to maintain strong incentives for cost efficiency by putting all of the managed care benefits at full risk while appropriately compensating plans that enroll a population with higher acuity. For Medicaid managed care programs that cover acute care services, several states have used diagnosis-based risk adjustment to control for the risk of high-cost populations, even after adjusting for such characteristics as enrollees' basis of Medicaid eligibility (e.g., disability). However, these commonly available risk adjustment models are based on health diagnostic data that are poor predictors of LTSS use (Davidson and Dreyfus 2012).

To address LTSS costs, most states use a variety of rate-setting design options such as defining relevant rate cells, making add-on payments, or allowing partial risk arrangements for the nursing facility benefit. Questions remain as to how well these different methodologies maintain incentives for plans to utilize the most cost-effective setting of care (Kronick and Llanos 2010).

As stated previously, only a few states currently have implemented an LTSS risk adjustment model. The creation of a public or commercial risk adjustment model for LTSS could make it easier for states to adopt capitated managed care approaches for LTSS users, including dual eligibles. There would be several challenges to developing such a model, however. Given the differences in the exact services states may include in their LTSS benefits package, a single model may not be predictive of LTSS costs across states.

Additionally, experience in risk adjustment for LTSS based on frailty and functional status has been limited, and the predictive power of such models has not been widely researched. The existing models may have limited predictive power in a given state, as that state may not be collecting information on the most predictive measures. Without widespread development and testing of different LTSS risk adjustment models, it will be difficult for a state to identify what additional measures it may want to collect to improve its model.

The financial alignment demonstrations provide an opportunity to review different risk adjustment models that states develop and identify what measures appear to be good predictors of LTSS costs across several states. These key predictors could serve as a foundation upon which other states could develop and enhance their own LTSS risk adjustment methodologies.

Need for measures of functional status

In order to develop and implement an LTSS risk adjustment process, relevant measures of frailty and functional status must be collected on a periodic basis. These measures are not typically found in Medicaid claims data, so they will likely require a separate assessment. In many states, the managed care plan is required to conduct a functional assessment to determine an enrollee's need for services and develop a care management plan when they first enroll. While these data could be used for risk adjustment, plans might have an incentive to "upcode" the frailty of their enrollees to receive higher capitation payments. States may need to validate the assessment data before using it for payment purposes.

Treatment of supplemental payments

As mentioned in MACPAC's June 2011 and March 2012 Reports to the Congress, states may make supplemental payments to institutional providers such as hospitals and nursing facilities, above what they pay for individual services. States make these supplemental payments under the federal UPL regulation.[10] These UPL supplemental payments may be a large source of revenue for institutional providers and have had important implications in states' decisions regarding managed care. Since the UPL supplemental payments are based on FFS days in an institutional setting, transitioning populations from FFS to managed care would lead to lower supplemental payments.

Additionally, these UPL supplemental payments cannot be included in the capitation rate or passed through the managed care plan to contracted providers because CMS considers these options to be inconsistent with the actuarial soundness principle. According to federal regulations, the services covered by Medicaid managed care plans must be considered paid in full through the rate paid to the plan (42 CFR 438.60). Some states have delayed implementation or expansion of Medicaid managed care because of the potential loss in federal matching dollars for supplemental payments. It is unclear whether these supplemental payments will be allowed to be included in the development of the Medicaid baseline for the financial alignment demonstration plans and may be an issue in some states.

Endnotes

1 Twenty states submitted proposals for the financial alignment capitated model; however, five states have recently indicated they will no longer pursue the capitated demonstration.

2 More information regarding the Medicare Advantage and Part D payment process can be found in the Medicare Payment Advisory Commission's *Payment basics* publications (MedPAC 2012a and 2012b).

3 The financial alignment demonstration will allow states to passively enroll dual eligibles into managed care plans, but beneficiaries will have the option to disenroll.

4 42 CFR 438.6(c) specifies that actuarially sound rates must be developed in accordance with generally accepted actuarial principles and practices and be certified by a qualified actuary. Capitation payment rates reflect only those services covered under the Medicaid state plan (or directly related costs such as administrative expenses) that are specified in the contract.

5 Massachusetts phased out the risk corridors in the SCO program in 2008.

6 42 CFR 460.150(d) specifies that eligibility to enroll in a PACE program is not restricted to an individual who is either a Medicare beneficiary or Medicaid enrollee. In practice, about 90 percent of all PACE enrollees are dual eligibles (Mathematica Policy Research analysis for MACPAC, 2012).

7 Actuarial soundness means that the capitation rates are developed in accordance with generally accepted actuarial principles and practices and certified by a qualified actuary.

8 Medicare Part A generally covers inpatient hospital services, skilled nursing facility services, and hospice care. Medicare Part B covers outpatient hospital, physician and other medical services such as laboratory, x-ray, and durable medical equipment. Medicare Part D covers outpatient prescription drugs.

9 CMS-HCC is the hierarchical condition category model currently used to risk adjust Medicare Advantage payments. RxHCC is the model of prescription drug hierarchical condition categories currently used to risk adjust Medicare Part D payments.

10 The UPL regulations governing payment to institutions limit total Medicaid payment to no more than what Medicare would have paid for the same or comparable services delivered by those same institutions. This UPL is different from the UPL established for PACE programs.

References

Arizona Health Care Cost Containment System Administration (AHCCCS). 2012. Section D.56. In *ALTCS EPD CY13, Contract Amendment*. Phoenix, AZ: Arizona Health Care Cost Containment System Administration. http://www.azahcccs.gov/commercial/Downloads/ContractAmendments/ALTCS/ALTCSCYE2012/CYE13ALTCSEPD.pdf.

Bella, M. 2012. Statement on Examining Medicare and Medicaid coordination for dual-eligibles before the Special Committee on Aging, U.S. Senate, July 18, 2012, Washington, DC. http://www.aging.senate.gov/hearing_detail.cfm?id=337279&.

Bella, M., and L. Palmer. 2009. *Encouraging integrated care for dual eligibles*. Hamilton, NJ: Center for Health Care Strategies, Inc. http://www.chcs.org/usr_doc/Integrated_Care_Resource_Paper.pdf.

Centers for Medicare & Medicaid Services (CMS), U.S. Department of Health and Human Services. 2013. *Joint rate-setting process under the capitated financial alignment initiative*. Washington, DC: CMS. http://www.cms.gov/Medicare-Medicaid-Coordination/Medicare-and-Medicaid-Coordination/Medicare-Medicaid-Coordination-Office/Downloads/JointRateSettingProcess.pdf.

Centers for Medicare & Medicaid Services (CMS), U.S. Department of Health and Human Services. 2012a. *Memorandum of Understanding (MOU) between the Centers for Medicare & Medicaid Services (CMS) and the Commonwealth of Massachusetts regarding a federal-state partnership to test a capitated financial alignment model for Medicare-Medicaid enrollees: Demonstration to integrate care for dual eligible beneficiaries*. Washington, DC: CMS. https://www.cms.gov/Medicare-Medicaid-Coordination/Medicare-and-Medicaid-Coordination/Medicare-Medicaid-Coordination-Office/Downloads/MassMOU.pdf.

Centers for Medicare & Medicaid Services (CMS), U.S. Department of Health and Human Services. 2012b. *Memorandum of Understanding (MOU) between the Centers for Medicare & Medicaid Services (CMS) and the state of Ohio regarding a federal-state partnership to test a capitated financial alignment model for Medicare-Medicaid enrollees: Demonstration to develop an integrated care delivery system*. Washington, DC: CMS. https://www.cms.gov/Medicare-Medicaid-Coordination/Medicare-and-Medicaid-Coordination/Medicare-Medicaid-Coordination-Office/Downloads/OHMOU.pdf.

Davidson, E.B. and T. Dreyfus. 2012. *Risk adjustment for dual eligibles: breaking new ground in Massachusetts.* Boston, MA: Massachusetts Medicaid Policy Institute. http://bluecrossmafoundation.org/sites/default/files/RiskAdjustment_Jan2012_v7.pdf.

Kronick, R. and K. Llanos. 2008. *Rate setting for Medicaid managed long-term supports and services: best practices and recommendations for states.* Hamilton, NJ: Center for Health Care Strategies, Inc. http://www.chcs.org/publications3960/publications_show.htm?doc_id=670910.

Massachusetts Department of Health and Human Services (DHHS). 2010. Section 4: Payment and financial provisions. In *MassHealth Senior Care Options—Contract for senior care organizations.* Boston, MA: Massachusetts Department of Health and Human Services. http://www.chcs.org/usr_doc/2010_contract.pdf.

Mathematica Policy Research. 2012. Analysis for MACPAC. Unpublished.

Medicaid and CHIP Payment and Access Commission (MACPAC). 2011. *Report to Congress: The evolution of managed care in Medicaid.* June 2011. Washington, DC: MACPAC. http://www.macpac.gov/reports.

Medicare Payment Advisory Commission (MedPAC). 2012a. *Medicare payment basics: Medicare Advantage program payment system.* Washington, DC: MedPAC. http://www.medpac.gov/documents/MedPAC_Payment_Basics_12_MA.pdf.

Medicare Payment Advisory Commission (MedPAC). 2012b. *Medicare payment basics: Part D payment system.* Washington, DC: MedPAC. http://www.medpac.gov/documents/MedPAC_Payment_Basiscs_12_PartD.pdf.

Minnesota Department of Human Services (DHS). 2012. Article 4.9.2, Payment for skilled nursing facility/nursing facility benefit. In *2012 MSHO/MSC+ Contract Model.* St. Paul, MN: Minnesota Department of Human Services. http://www.dhs.state.mn.us/main/groups/business_partners/documents/pub/dhs16_166538.pdf.

National PACE Association. 2012. *PACE in the states.* October 2012. http://www.npaonline.org/website/navdispatch.asp?id=1741.

National PACE Association. 2009. *PACE Medicaid rate-setting: Issues and considerations for states and PACE organizations.* May 2009. http://www.npaonline.org/website/navdispatch.asp?id=2871.

Saucier, P., J. Kasten, B. Burwell, et al. 2012. *The growth of managed long-term services and supports (MLTSS) programs: A 2012 update.* Report to CMS, contract no. HHSM-500-2005-000251. July 2012. Ann Arbor, MI: Truven Health Analytics. http://www.medicaid.gov/Medicaid-CHIP-Program-Information/By-Topics/Delivery-Systems/Downloads/MLTSSP_White_paper_combined.pdf.

Texas Health & Human Services Commission (HHSC). 2012. Attachment B-1 Section 6. In *STAR+PLUS expansion contract - version 1.8.* Austin, TX: Texas Health and Human Services Commission. http://www.hhsc.state.tx.us/medicaid/STARPLUSExpansionContract.pdf.

Wisconsin Department of Health Services (DHS). 2012. *Calendar Year 2012 Program of All Inclusive Care for the Elderly (PACE) and Family Care Partnership Program (FCP) managed care equivalent values.* Madison, WI: Wisconsin Department of Health Services. January 2012. http://www.dhs.wisconsin.gov/LTCare/StateFedReqs/ratereport2012fcp.pdf.

Appendix

Acronym List

ACA	Patient Protection and Affordable Care Act
ADL	Activities of Daily Living
AFDC	Aid to Families with Dependent Children
AHA	American Hospital Association
AHCA	American Health Care Association
ARRA	American Recovery and Reinvestment Act
BBA	Balanced Budget Act
CBO	Congressional Budget Office
CHIP	State Children's Health Insurance Program
CHIPRA	Children's Health Insurance Program Reauthorization Act
CMS	Centers for Medicare & Medicaid Services
DME	Durable Medical Equipment
DRA	Deficit Reduction Act
DSH	Disproportionate Share Hospital
D-SNP	Dual-eligible Special Needs Plan
E-FMAP	Enhanced Federal Medical Assistance Percentage
EPSDT	Early and Periodic Screening, Diagnostic, and Treatment
ESI	Employer-sponsored Insurance
FFP	Federal Financial Participation
FFS	Fee for Service
FIDE SNP	Fully Integrated Dual-eligible Special Needs Plan
FMAP	Federal Medical Assistance Percentage
FMR	Financial Management Report
FPL	Federal Poverty Level
FY	Fiscal Year
GAO	U.S. Government Accountability Office
HCBS	Home and Community-based Services
HCC	Hierarchical Condition Categories
HCFA	Health Care Financing Administration
HCRP	High Cost Risk Pool
HHS	U.S. Department of Health and Human Services

ICF/ID	Intermediate Care Facility for Persons with Intellectual Disabilities
IHS	Indian Health Service
IRS	Internal Revenue Service
KFF	Kaiser Family Foundation
LIS	Low-income Subsidy
LTSS	Long-term Services and Supports
MAGI	Modified Adjusted Gross Income
MAX	Medicaid Analytic eXtract
MBES/CBES	Medicaid and CHIP Budget Expenditure System
MCCA	Medicare Catastrophic Coverage Act
MCO	Managed Care Organization
MEMA	Member Enrollment Mix Adjustment
MIPPA	Medicare Improvements for Patients and Providers Act
MMCO	Medicare-Medicaid Coordination Office
MMLR	Minimum Medical Loss Ratio
MOE	Maintenance of Effort
MOU	Memorandum of Understanding
MSHO	Minnesota Senior Health Options
MSIS	Medicaid Statistical Information System
MSP	Medicare Savings Program
NASBO	National Association of State Budget Officers
NFIB	National Federation of Independent Business
NFLOC	Nursing Facility Level of Care
NHE	National Health Expenditures
NHIS	National Health Interview Survey
OACT	Office of the Actuary
OBRA	Omnibus Budget Reconciliation Act
OHCA	Oklahoma Health Care Authority
OIG	Office of Inspector General
PACE	Program of All-inclusive Care for the Elderly
PCCM	Primary Care Case Management
PCP	Primary Care Provider
PPS	Prospective Payment System
QDWI	Qualifying Disabled and Working Individual
QI	Qualifying Individual
QMB	Qualified Medicare Beneficiary
SCO	Senior Care Options

SEDS	Statistical Enrollment Data System
SIPP	Survey of Income and Program Participation
SLMB	Specified Low-income Medicare Beneficiary
SNF	Skilled Nursing Facility
SNP	Special Needs Plan
SSA	U.S. Social Security Administration
SSDI	Social Security Disability Insurance
SSI	Supplemental Security Income
TANF	Temporary Assistance for Needy Families
TEFRA	Tax Equity and Fiscal Responsibility Act
TMA	Transitional Medical Assistance
UPL	Upper Payment Limit
VFC	Vaccines for Children

Authorizing Language from the Social Security Act (42 U.S.C. 1396)

MEDICAID AND CHIP PAYMENT AND ACCESS COMMISSION

(a) ESTABLISHMENT.—There is hereby established the Medicaid and CHIP Payment and Access Commission (in this section referred to as 'MACPAC').

(b) DUTIES.—

(1) REVIEW OF ACCESS POLICIES FOR ALL STATES AND ANNUAL REPORTS.—MACPAC shall—

(A) review policies of the Medicaid program established under this title (in this section referred to as 'Medicaid') and the State Children's Health Insurance Program established under title XXI (in this section referred to as 'CHIP') affecting access to covered items and services, including topics described in paragraph (2);

(B) make recommendations to Congress, the Secretary, and States concerning such access policies;

(C) by not later than March 15 of each year (beginning with 2010), submit a report to Congress containing the results of such reviews and MACPAC's recommendations concerning such policies; and

(D) by not later than June 15 of each year (beginning with 2010), submit a report to Congress containing an examination of issues affecting Medicaid and CHIP, including the implications of changes in health care delivery in the United States and in the market for health care services on such programs.

(2) SPECIFIC TOPICS TO BE REVIEWED.—Specifically, MACPAC shall review and assess the following:

(A) MEDICAID AND CHIP PAYMENT POLICIES.—Payment policies under Medicaid and CHIP, including—

(i) the factors affecting expenditures for the efficient provision of items and services in different sectors, including the process for updating payments to medical, dental, and health professionals, hospitals, residential and long-term care providers, providers of home and community based services, Federally-qualified health centers and rural health clinics, managed care entities, and providers of other covered items and services;

(ii) payment methodologies; and

(iii) the relationship of such factors and methodologies to access and quality of care for Medicaid and CHIP beneficiaries (including how such factors and methodologies enable such beneficiaries to obtain the services for which they are eligible, affect provider supply, and affect providers that serve a disproportionate share of low-income and other vulnerable populations).

(B) ELIGIBILITY POLICIES.—Medicaid and CHIP eligibility policies, including a determination of the degree to which Federal and State policies provide health care coverage to needy populations.

(C) ENROLLMENT AND RETENTION PROCESSES.—Medicaid and CHIP enrollment and retention processes, including a determination of the degree to which Federal and State policies encourage the enrollment of individuals who are eligible for such programs and screen out individuals who are ineligible, while minimizing the share of program expenses devoted to such processes.

(D) COVERAGE POLICIES.—Medicaid and CHIP benefit and coverage policies, including a determination of the degree to which Federal and State policies provide access to the services enrollees require to improve and maintain their health and functional status.

(E) QUALITY OF CARE.—Medicaid and CHIP policies as they relate to the quality of care provided under those programs, including a determination of the degree to which Federal and State policies achieve their stated goals and interact with similar goals established by other purchasers of health care services.

(F) INTERACTION OF MEDICAID AND CHIP PAYMENT POLICIES WITH HEALTH CARE DELIVERY GENERALLY.—The effect of Medicaid and CHIP payment policies on access to items and services for children and other Medicaid and CHIP populations other than under this title or title XXI and the implications of changes in health care delivery in the United States and in the general market for health care items and services on Medicaid and CHIP.

(G) INTERACTIONS WITH MEDICARE AND MEDICAID.—Consistent with paragraph (11), the interaction of policies under Medicaid and the Medicare program under title XVIII, including with respect to how such interactions affect access to services, payments, and dual eligible individuals.

(H) OTHER ACCESS POLICIES.—The effect of other Medicaid and CHIP policies on access to covered items and services, including policies relating to transportation and language barriers and preventive, acute, and long-term services and supports.

(3) RECOMMENDATIONS AND REPORTS OF STATE-SPECIFIC DATA.—MACPAC shall—

(A) review national and State-specific Medicaid and CHIP data; and

(B) submit reports and recommendations to Congress, the Secretary, and States based on such reviews.

(4) CREATION OF EARLY-WARNING SYSTEM.—MACPAC shall create an early-warning system to identify provider shortage areas, as well as other factors that adversely affect, or have the potential to adversely affect, access to care by, or the health care status of, Medicaid and CHIP beneficiaries. MACPAC shall include in the annual report required under paragraph (1)(D) a description of all such areas or problems identified with respect to the period addressed in the report.

(5) COMMENTS ON CERTAIN SECRETARIAL REPORTS AND REGULATIONS.—

(A) CERTAIN SECRETARIAL REPORTS.—If the Secretary submits to Congress (or a committee of Congress) a report that is required by law and that relates to access policies, including with respect to payment policies, under Medicaid or CHIP, the Secretary shall transmit a copy of the report to MACPAC. MACPAC shall review the report and, not later than 6 months after the date of submittal of the Secretary's report to Congress, shall submit to the appropriate committees of Congress and the Secretary written comments on such report. Such comments may include such recommendations as MACPAC deems appropriate.

(B) REGULATIONS.—MACPAC shall review Medicaid and CHIP regulations and may comment through submission of a report to the appropriate committees of Congress and the Secretary, on any such regulations that affect access, quality, or efficiency of health care.

(6) AGENDA AND ADDITIONAL REVIEWS.—MACPAC shall consult periodically with the chairmen and ranking minority members of the appropriate committees of Congress regarding MACPAC's agenda and progress towards achieving the agenda. MACPAC may conduct additional reviews, and submit additional reports to the appropriate committees of Congress, from time to time on such topics relating to the program under this title or title XXI as may be requested by such chairmen and members and as MACPAC deems appropriate.

(7) AVAILABILITY OF REPORTS.—MACPAC shall transmit to the Secretary a copy of each report submitted under this subsection and shall make such reports available to the public.

(8) APPROPRIATE COMMITTEE OF CONGRESS.—For purposes of this section, the term 'appropriate committees of Congress' means the Committee on Energy and Commerce of the House of Representatives and the Committee on Finance of the Senate.

(9) VOTING AND REPORTING REQUIREMENTS.—With respect to each recommendation contained in a report submitted under paragraph (1), each member of MACPAC shall vote on the recommendation, and MACPAC shall include, by member, the results of that vote in the report containing the recommendation.

(10) EXAMINATION OF BUDGET CONSEQUENCES.—Before making any recommendations, MACPAC shall examine the budget consequences of such recommendations, directly or through consultation with appropriate expert entities, and shall submit with any recommendations, a report on the Federal and State-specific budget consequences of the recommendations.

(11) CONSULTATION AND COORDINATION WITH MEDPAC.—

(A) IN GENERAL.—MACPAC shall consult with the Medicare Payment Advisory Commission (in this paragraph referred to as 'MedPAC') established under section 1805 in carrying out its duties under this section, as appropriate and particularly with respect to the issues specified in paragraph (2) as they relate to those Medicaid beneficiaries who are dually eligible for Medicaid and the Medicare program under title XVIII, adult Medicaid beneficiaries (who are not dually eligible for Medicare), and beneficiaries under Medicare. Responsibility for analysis of and recommendations to change Medicare policy regarding Medicare beneficiaries, including Medicare beneficiaries who are dually eligible for Medicare and Medicaid, shall rest with MedPAC.

(B) INFORMATION SHARING.—MACPAC and MedPAC shall have access to deliberations and records of the other such entity, respectively, upon the request of the other such entity.

(12) CONSULTATION WITH STATES.—MACPAC shall regularly consult with States in carrying out its duties under this section, including with respect to developing processes for carrying out such duties, and shall ensure that input from States is taken into account and represented in MACPAC's recommendations and reports.

(13) COORDINATE AND CONSULT WITH THE FEDERAL COORDINATED HEALTH CARE OFFICE.—MACPAC shall coordinate and consult with the Federal Coordinated Health Care Office established under section 2081 of the Patient Protection and Affordable Care Act before making any recommendations regarding dual eligible individuals.

(14) PROGRAMMATIC OVERSIGHT VESTED IN THE SECRETARY.— MACPAC's authority to make recommendations in accordance with this section shall not affect, or be considered to duplicate, the Secretary's authority to carry out Federal responsibilities with respect to Medicaid and CHIP.

(c) MEMBERSHIP.—

(1) NUMBER AND APPOINTMENT.—MACPAC shall be composed of 17 members appointed by the Comptroller General of the United States.

(2) QUALIFICATIONS.—

(A) IN GENERAL.—The membership of MACPAC shall include individuals who have had direct experience as enrollees or parents or caregivers of enrollees in Medicaid or CHIP and individuals with national recognition for their expertise in Federal safety net health programs, health finance and economics, actuarial science, health plans and integrated delivery systems, reimbursement for health care, health information technology, and other providers of health services, public health, and other related fields, who provide a mix of different professions, broad geographic representation, and a balance between urban and rural representation.

(B) INCLUSION.—The membership of MACPAC shall include (but not be limited to) physicians, dentists, and other health professionals, employers, third-party payers, and individuals with expertise in the delivery of health services. Such membership shall also include representatives of children, pregnant women, the elderly, individuals with disabilities, caregivers, and dual eligible individuals, current or former representatives of State agencies responsible for administering Medicaid, and current or former representatives of State agencies responsible for administering CHIP.

(C) MAJORITY NONPROVIDERS.—Individuals who are directly involved in the provision, or management of the delivery, of items and services covered under Medicaid or CHIP shall not constitute a majority of the membership of MACPAC.

(D) ETHICAL DISCLOSURE.—The Comptroller General of the United States shall establish a system for public disclosure by members of MACPAC of financial and other potential conflicts of interest relating to such members. Members of MACPAC shall be treated as employees of Congress for purposes of applying title I of the Ethics in Government Act of 1978 (Public Law 95–521).

(3) TERMS.—

(A) IN GENERAL.—The terms of members of MACPAC shall be for 3 years except that the Comptroller General of the United States shall designate staggered terms for the members first appointed.

(B) VACANCIES.—Any member appointed to fill a vacancy occurring before the expiration of the term for which the member's predecessor was appointed shall be appointed only for the remainder of that term. A member may serve after the expiration of that member's term until a successor has taken office. A vacancy in MACPAC shall be filled in the manner in which the original appointment was made.

(4) COMPENSATION.—While serving on the business of MACPAC (including travel time), a member of MACPAC shall be entitled to compensation at the per diem equivalent of the rate provided for level IV of the Executive Schedule under section 5315 of title 5, United States Code; and while so serving away from home and the member's regular place of business, a member may be allowed travel expenses, as authorized by the Chairman of MACPAC. Physicians serving as personnel of MACPAC may be provided a physician comparability allowance by MACPAC in the same manner as Government physicians may be provided such an allowance by an agency under section 5948 of title 5, United States Code, and for such purpose subsection (i) of such section shall apply to MACPAC in the same manner as it applies to the Tennessee Valley Authority. For purposes of pay (other than pay of members of MACPAC) and employment benefits, rights, and privileges, all personnel of MACPAC shall be treated as if they were employees of the United States Senate.

(5) CHAIRMAN; VICE CHAIRMAN.—The Comptroller General of the United States shall designate a member of MACPAC, at the time of appointment of the member as Chairman and a member as Vice Chairman for that term of appointment, except that in the case of vacancy of the Chairmanship or Vice Chairmanship, the Comptroller General of the United States may designate another member for the remainder of that member's term.

(6) MEETINGS.—MACPAC shall meet at the call of the Chairman.

(d) DIRECTOR AND STAFF; EXPERTS AND CONSULTANTS.—Subject to such review as the Comptroller General of the United States deems necessary to assure the efficient administration of MACPAC, MACPAC may—

(1) employ and fix the compensation of an Executive Director (subject to the approval of the Comptroller General of the United States) and such other personnel as may be necessary to carry out its duties (without regard to the provisions of title 5, United States Code, governing appointments in the competitive service);

(2) seek such assistance and support as may be required in the performance of its duties from appropriate Federal and State departments and agencies;

(3) enter into contracts or make other arrangements, as may be necessary for the conduct of the work of MACPAC (without regard to section 3709 of the Revised Statutes (41 U.S.C. 5));

(4) make advance, progress, and other payments which relate to the work of MACPAC;

(5) provide transportation and subsistence for persons serving without compensation; and

(6) prescribe such rules and regulations as it deems necessary with respect to the internal organization and operation of MACPAC.

(e) POWERS.—

(1) OBTAINING OFFICIAL DATA.—MACPAC may secure directly from any department or agency of the United States and, as a condition for receiving payments under sections 1903(a) and 2105(a), from any State agency responsible for administering Medicaid or CHIP, information necessary to enable it to carry out this section. Upon request of the Chairman, the head of that department or agency shall furnish that information to MACPAC on an agreed upon schedule.

(2) DATA COLLECTION.—In order to carry out its functions, MACPAC shall—

(A) utilize existing information, both published and unpublished, where possible, collected and assessed either by its own staff or under other arrangements made in accordance with this section;

(B) carry out, or award grants or contracts for, original research and experimentation, where existing information is inadequate; and

(C) adopt procedures allowing any interested party to submit information for MACPAC's use in making reports and recommendations.

(3) ACCESS OF GAO TO INFORMATION.—The Comptroller General of the United States shall have unrestricted access to all deliberations, records, and nonproprietary data of MACPAC, immediately upon request.

(4) PERIODIC AUDIT.—MACPAC shall be subject to periodic audit by the Comptroller General of the United States.

(f) FUNDING.—

(1) REQUEST FOR APPROPRIATIONS.—MACPAC shall submit requests for appropriations (other than for fiscal year 2010) in the same manner as the Comptroller General of the United States submits requests for appropriations, but amounts appropriated for MACPAC shall be separate from amounts appropriated for the Comptroller General of the United States.

(2) AUTHORIZATION.—There are authorized to be appropriated such sums as may be necessary to carry out the provisions of this section.

(3) FUNDING FOR FISCAL YEAR 2010.—

(A) IN GENERAL.—Out of any funds in the Treasury not otherwise appropriated, there is appropriated to MACPAC to carry out the provisions of this section for fiscal year 2010, $9,000,000.

(B) TRANSFER OF FUNDS.—Notwithstanding section 2104(a)(13), from the amounts appropriated in such section for fiscal year 2010, $2,000,000 is hereby transferred and made available in such fiscal year to MACPAC to carry out the provisions of this section.

(4) AVAILABILITY.—Amounts made available under paragraphs (2) and (3) to MACPAC to carry out the provisions of this section shall remain available until expended.

Commission Votes on Recommendations

In its authorizing language in the Social Security Act (42 U.S.C. 1396), the Congress required MACPAC to review Medicaid and CHIP program policies and to make recommendations to the Congress, the Secretary of the U.S. Department of Health and Human Services, and the states related to those policies in its report due to the Congress by March 15 of each year. Each Commissioner must vote on each recommendation, and the votes for each recommendation must be published in the report. The recommendations included in this report and the corresponding voting record below fulfill this mandate.

Eligibility Issues in Medicaid and CHIP: Interactions with the ACA

2.1 In order to ensure that current eligibility options remain available to states in 2014, the Congress should, parallel to the existing Medicaid 12-month continuous eligibility option for children, create a similar statutory option for children enrolled in CHIP and adults enrolled in Medicaid.

14 Yes
0 No
0 Not Voting
3 Not Present

Yes: Carte, Chambers, Cohen, Edelstein, Gabow, Henning, Hoyt, Martínez Rogers, Moore, Riley, Rosenbaum, Rowland, Smith, Waldren

Not Present: Checkett, Gray, Sundwall

Eligibility Issues in Medicaid and CHIP: Interactions with the ACA

2.2 The Congress should permanently fund current Transitional Medical Assistance (TMA) (required for six months, with state option for 12 months), while allowing states to opt out of TMA if they expand to the new adult group added under the Patient Protection and Affordable Care Act.

14 Yes
0 No
0 Not Voting
3 Not Present

Yes: Carte, Chambers, Cohen, Edelstein, Gabow, Henning, Hoyt, Martínez Rogers, Moore, Riley, Rosenbaum, Rowland, Smith, Waldren

Not Present: Checkett, Gray, Sundwall

Biographies of Commissioners

Sharon L. Carte, M.H.S., is executive director of the West Virginia Children's Health Insurance Program. From 1992 to 1998, Ms. Carte served as the deputy commissioner for the Bureau for Medical Services overseeing West Virginia's Medicaid program. Prior to that, she was administrator of skilled and intermediate care nursing facilities and before that a coordinator of human resources development in the West Virginia Department of Health. Ms. Carte has also worked with senior centers and aging programs throughout the State of West Virginia and on policies related to behavioral health and chronic care for children with mental illness. She received her master of health science from The Johns Hopkins University.

Richard Chambers is president of Molina Healthcare of California, a health plan serving 345,000 Medicaid, CHIP, and Medicare Advantage Special Needs Plan (SNP) members in five counties in California. Nationally, Molina Healthcare arranges for the delivery of health care services or offers health information management solutions for nearly 4.2 million individuals and families who receive their care through Medicaid, CHIP, Medicare Advantage, and other government-funded programs in 15 states. Before joining Molina Healthcare in 2012, Mr. Chambers was chief executive officer for nine years at CalOptima, a County Organized Health System providing health coverage to 410,000 low-income residents in Orange County, California, through Medicaid, CHIP, and Medicare Advantage SNP programs. Prior to CalOptima, Mr. Chambers spent over 27 years working for the Centers for Medicare & Medicaid Services (CMS). He served as the director of the Family and Children's Health Programs Group, responsible for national policy and operational direction of Medicaid and CHIP. While at CMS, Mr. Chambers also served as associate regional administrator for Medicaid in the San Francisco Regional Office and as director of the Office of Intergovernmental Affairs in the Washington, DC office. He received his bachelor's degree from the University of Virginia.

Donna Checkett, M.P.A., M.S.W., is vice president of state government relations at Aetna. Prior to that, she was the chief executive officer of Missouri Care, a managed Medicaid health plan owned by University of Missouri-Columbia Health Care, one of the largest safety net hospital systems in the state. For eight years, Ms. Checkett served as the director of the Missouri Division of Medical Services (Medicaid), during which time she was the chair of the National Association of State Medicaid Directors and a member of the National Governors Association Medicaid Improvements Working Group. She served as chair of the Advisory Board for the Center for Health Care Strategies, a non-profit health policy resource center dedicated to improving health care quality for low-income children and adults. Ms. Checkett also served as chair of the National Advisory Committee for Covering Kids, a Robert Wood Johnson Foundation program fostering outreach and eligibility simplification efforts for Medicaid and CHIP beneficiaries. She received her master of public administration from the University of Missouri-Columbia and a master of social work from the University of Texas at Austin.

Andrea Cohen, J.D., is the director of health services in the New York City Office of the

Mayor, where she coordinates and develops strategies to improve public health and health care services for New Yorkers. She serves on the board of the Primary Care Development Corporation and represents the deputy mayor for health and human services on the Board of the Health and Hospitals Corporation, the largest public hospital system in the country. From 2005 to 2009, Ms. Cohen was counsel with Manatt, Phelps & Phillips, LLP, where she advised clients on issues relating to Medicare, Medicaid, and other public health insurance programs. Prior professional positions include senior policy counsel at the Medicare Rights Center, health and oversight counsel for the U.S. Senate Committee on Finance, and attorney with the U.S. Department of Justice. She received her law degree from Columbia University School of Law.

Burton L. Edelstein, D.D.S., M.P.H., is a board-certified pediatric dentist and professor of dentistry and health policy and management at Columbia University. He is founding president of the Children's Dental Health Project, a national non-profit Washington, DC-based policy organization that promotes equity in children's oral health. Dr. Edelstein practiced pediatric dentistry in Connecticut and taught at the Harvard School of Dental Medicine for 21 years prior to serving as a 1996–1997 Robert Wood Johnson Foundation health policy fellow in the office of U.S. Senate leader Tom Daschle, with primary responsibility for the State Children's Health Insurance Program (S-CHIP). Dr. Edelstein worked with the U.S. Department of Health and Human Services on its oral health initiatives from 1998 to 2001, chaired the U.S. Surgeon General's Workshop on Children and Oral Health, and authored the child section of *Oral Health in America: A Report of the Surgeon General*. His research focuses on children's oral health promotion and access to dental care with a particular emphasis on Medicaid and CHIP populations. He received his degree in dentistry from the State University of New York at Buffalo School of Dentistry, his master of public health from Harvard University School of Public Health, and completed his clinical training at Boston Children's Hospital.

Patricia Gabow, M.D., was chief executive officer of Denver Health from 1992 until her retirement in 2012, transforming it from a department of city government to a successful, independent governmental entity. She is a member of the Commonwealth Commission on a High Performance Health System, the Institute of Medicine (IOM) Roundtable on Value and Science Driven Health Care, and the National Governors Association Health Advisory Board. Dr. Gabow is a professor of medicine at the University of Colorado School of Medicine and has authored over 150 articles and book chapters. She received her medical degree from the University of Pennsylvania School of Medicine. Dr. Gabow has received the American Medical Association's Nathan Davis Award for Outstanding Public Servant, the Ohtli Award from the Mexican government, the National Healthcare Leadership Award, the David E. Rogers Award from the Association of American Medical Colleges, the Health Quality Leader Award from the National Committee for Quality Assurance (NCQA), and election to the Association for Manufacturing Excellence Hall of Fame for her work on Toyota Production Systems in health care.

Herman Gray, M.D., M.B.A., is president of Children's Hospital of Michigan (CHM) and senior vice president of the Detroit Medical Center. At CHM, Dr. Gray served previously as pediatrics vice chief for education, director of the Pediatric Residency Program, chief of staff, and then chief operating officer. He also served as associate dean for graduate medical education (GME) and vice president for GME at Wayne State University School of Medicine and the Detroit Medical

Center, respectively. Dr. Gray has also served as the chief medical consultant for the Michigan Department of Public Health Division of Children's Special Health Care Services and as vice president and medical director of clinical affairs for Blue Care Network. During the 1980s, he pursued private medical practice in Detroit. Dr. Gray serves on the board of trustees of the National Association of Children's Hospitals and the board of directors of the Child Health Corporation of America, now merged and known as Children's Hospital Association. He received his medical degree from the University of Michigan in Ann Arbor, and a master of business administration from the University of Tennessee.

Denise Henning, C.N.M., M.S.N., is clinical director for women's health at Collier Health Services, a federally qualified health center in Immokalee, Florida. A practicing nurse-midwife, Ms. Henning provides prenatal and gynecological care to a service population that is predominantly either uninsured or covered by Medicaid. From 2003 to 2008, she was director of clinical operations for Women's Health Services at the Family Health Centers of Southwest Florida, where she supervised the midwifery and other clinical staff. Prior to this, Ms. Henning served as a certified nurse-midwife in several locations in Florida and as a labor and delivery nurse in a Level III teaching hospital. She is a former president of the Midwifery Business Network and chair of the business section of the American College of Nurse-Midwives. She received her master of science in nurse-midwifery from the University of Florida in Jacksonville and her bachelor of science in nursing from the University of Florida in Gainesville. She also holds a degree in business management from Nova University in Fort Lauderdale, Florida.

Mark Hoyt, F.S.A., M.A.A.A., was the national practice leader of the Government Human Services Consulting group of Mercer Health & Benefits, LLC until his retirement in 2012. This group helps states purchase health services for their Medicaid and CHIP programs and has worked with over 30 states. He joined Mercer in 1980 and worked on government health care projects starting in 1987, including developing strategies for statewide health reform, evaluating the impact of different managed care approaches, and overseeing program design and rate analysis for Medicaid and CHIP programs. Mr. Hoyt is a fellow in the Society of Actuaries and a member of the American Academy of Actuaries. He received a master of arts in mathematics from the University of California at Berkeley.

Judith Moore is an independent consultant specializing in policy related to health, vulnerable populations, and social safety net issues. Ms. Moore's expertise in Medicaid, Medicare, long-term services and supports, and other state and federal programs flows from her career as a federal senior executive who served in the legislative and executive branches of government. At the Health Care Financing Administration (now the Centers for Medicare & Medicaid Services), Ms. Moore served as director of the Medicaid program and of the Office of Legislation and Congressional Affairs. Her federal service was followed by more than a decade as co-director and senior fellow at George Washington University's National Health Policy Forum, a non-partisan education program serving federal legislative and regulatory health staff. In addition to other papers and research, she is co-author with David G. Smith of a political history of Medicaid: *Medicaid Politics and Policy*.

Trish Riley, M.S., is an adjunct professor of health policy and management at the Muskie School of Public Service, University of Southern Maine and was the first distinguished visiting fellow and lecturer in state health policy at The George Washington University, following her tenure as director of the Maine Governor's Office of Health Policy and Finance. She was a principal architect of the Dirigo Health Reform Act of 2003, which was enacted to increase access, reduce costs, and improve quality of health care in Maine. Ms. Riley previously served as executive director of the National Academy for State Health Policy and as president of its Corporate Board. Under four Maine governors, she held appointed positions including executive director of the Maine Committee on Aging; director of the Bureau of Maine's Elderly; associate deputy commissioner of health and medical services; and director of the Bureau of Medical Services, responsible for the Medicaid program, and health planning and licensure. Ms. Riley served on Maine's Commission on Children's Health, which planned the S-CHIP program. She is a member of the Kaiser Commission on Medicaid and the Uninsured and has served as a member of the IOM's Subcommittee on Creating an External Environment for Quality and its Subcommittee on Maximizing the Value of Health. Ms. Riley has also served as a member of the board of directors of the NCQA. She received her master of science in community development from the University of Maine.

Norma Martínez Rogers, Ph.D., R.N., F.A.A.N., is a professor of family nursing at the University of Texas (UT) Health Science Center at San Antonio, where she has served on the faculty since 1996. Dr. Martínez Rogers has held clinical and administrative positions in psychiatric nursing and at psychiatric hospitals, including the William Beaumont Army Medical Center in Fort Bliss during Operation Desert Storm. She has initiated a number of programs at the UT Health Science Center in San Antonio, including a support group for women transitioning from prison back into society and the Martínez Street Women's Center, a non-profit organization designed to provide support and educational services to women and teenage girls. Dr. Martínez Rogers is a fellow of the American Academy of Nursing and is the former president of the National Association of Hispanic Nurses. She received a master of science in psychiatric nursing from the UT Health Science Center at San Antonio and her doctorate in cultural foundations in education from the UT at Austin.

Sara Rosenbaum, J.D., is founding chair of the Department of Health Policy and the Harold and Jane Hirsh Professor of Health Law and Policy at the George Washington (GW) University School of Public Health and Health Services. She also serves on the faculties of the GW Schools of Law and Medicine. Professor Rosenbaum's research has focused on how the law intersects with the nation's health care and public health systems, with a particular emphasis on insurance coverage, managed care, the health care safety net, health care quality, and civil rights. She is a member of the IOM and has served on the boards of numerous national organizations, including AcademyHealth. Professor Rosenbaum is a member of the Centers for Disease Control and Prevention's (CDC) Advisory Committee on Immunization Practices and also serves on the CDC Director's Advisory Committee. She has advised the Congress and presidential administrations since 1977 and served on the staff of the White House Domestic Policy Council during the Clinton Administration. Professor Rosenbaum is the leading author of *Law and the American Health Care System*, published by Foundation Press (2012). She received her law degree from Boston University School of Law.

Diane Rowland, Sc.D., has served as chair of MACPAC since December 2009. She is the executive vice president of the Henry J. Kaiser Family Foundation and the executive director of the Kaiser Commission on Medicaid and the Uninsured. She is also an adjunct professor in the Department of Health Policy and Management at the Johns Hopkins Bloomberg School of Public Health. Dr. Rowland has directed the Kaiser Commission since 1991 and has overseen the foundation's health policy work since 1993. She is a noted authority on health policy, Medicare and Medicaid, and health care for low-income and disadvantaged populations, and she frequently testifies as an expert witness before the U.S. Congress on health policy issues. A nationally recognized expert with a distinguished career in public policy and research, focusing on health insurance coverage, access to care, and health care financing for low-income, elderly, and disabled populations, Dr. Rowland has published widely on these subjects. She is an elected member of the IOM, a founding member of the National Academy for Social Insurance, past president and fellow of the Association for Health Services Research (now AcademyHealth), and a member of the board of Grantmakers In Health. Dr. Rowland holds a bachelor's degree from Wellesley College, a master of public administration from the University of California at Los Angeles, and a doctor of science in health policy and management from The Johns Hopkins University.

Robin Smith and her husband Doug have been foster and adoptive parents for many children covered by Medicaid, including many children with special needs. Her experience seeking care for these children has included working with an interdisciplinary Medicaid program called the Medically Fragile Children's Program, a national model partnership between the Medical University of South Carolina Children's Hospital, South Carolina Medicaid, and the South Carolina Department of Social Services. Ms. Smith serves on the Family Advisory Committee for the Children's Hospital at the Medical University of South Carolina. She has testified at congressional briefings and presented at the 2007 International Conference of Family Centered Care and at grand rounds for medical students and residents at the Medical University of South Carolina.

David Sundwall, M.D., serves as vice chair of MACPAC. He is a clinical professor of public health at the University of Utah School of Medicine, Division of Public Health, where he has been a faculty member since 1978. He served as executive director of the Utah Department of Health and commissioner of health for the State of Utah from 2005 through 2010. He currently serves on numerous government and community boards and advisory groups in his home state, including as chair of the Utah State Controlled Substance Advisory Committee. Dr. Sundwall was president of the Association of State and Territorial Health Officials from 2007 to 2008. He has chaired or served on several committees of the IOM and is currently on the IOM Committee on Integrating Primary Care and Public Health, and the Standing Committee on Health Threats Resilience. Prior to returning to Utah in 2005, he was president of the American Clinical Laboratory Association and before that was vice president and medical director of American Healthcare Systems. Dr. Sundwall's federal government experience includes serving as administrator of the Health Resources and Services Administration, assistant surgeon general in the Commissioned Corps of the U.S. Public Health Service, and director of the health and human resources staff of the Senate Labor and Human Resources Committee. He received his medical degree from the University of Utah School of Medicine, and completed his residency in the Harvard Family Medicine Program. He is a licensed physician, board certified in internal medicine and family practice, and volunteers in a public health clinic one-half day each week.

Steven Waldren, M.D., M.S., is senior strategist for health information technology at the American Academy of Family Physicians. He also serves as vice chair of the American Society for Testing Materials' E31 Health Information Standards Committee. Dr. Waldren sits on several advisory boards dealing with health care information technology (IT), and he was a past co-chair of the Physicians Electronic Health Record Coalition, a group of more than 20 professional medical associations addressing issues around health IT. He received his medical degree from the University of Kansas School of Medicine. While completing a post-doctoral National Library of Medicine medical informatics fellowship, he completed a master of science in health care informatics from the University of Missouri, Columbia. Dr. Waldren is a co-founder in two start-ups dealing with health IT systems design: Open Health Data Inc. and New Health Networks LLC.

Biographies of Staff

Amy Bernstein, Sc.D., M.H.S.A., is senior advisor for research. She manages and provides oversight and guidance for all MACPAC research, data, and analysis projects, including statements of work, research plans, and all deliverables and products. She also directs analyses on Medicaid dental and maternity care policies. Her previous positions have included director of the Analytic Studies Branch at the Centers for Disease Control/National Center for Health Statistics, and senior analyst positions at the Alpha Center, the Prospective Payment Assessment Commission, the National Cancer Institute, and the Agency for Healthcare Research and Quality. Dr. Bernstein earned a master of health services administration degree from the University of Michigan School of Public Health and a doctor of science degree from the School of Hygiene and Public Health at The Johns Hopkins University.

Mathew Chase is chief information officer. He is responsible for the technology strategy, information architecture, security, and operations at MACPAC. Mr. Chase previously served as the information technology (IT) manager for the Medicare Payment Advisory Commission (MedPAC) from 2004 to 2005 where he was responsible for all aspects of technology: strategic planning, budget, security, data reliability, support, and administration. Mr. Chase has also provided IT expertise and leadership in the private sector to organizations such as Cirque du Soleil, *The Las Vegas Review-Journal,* and several internet start-ups. He received his bachelor of science degree in decision sciences and management information systems from George Mason University.

Benjamin Finder, M.P.H., is a senior analyst. His work focuses on benefits and payment policy. Prior to joining MACPAC, he served as an associate director in the Health Care Policy and Research Administration at the District of Columbia Department of Health Care Finance, and as an analyst at the Kaiser Family Foundation. Mr. Finder holds a master of public health degree from The George Washington University, where he concentrated in health policy and health economics.

Moira Forbes, M.B.A., is director of payment and program integrity, focusing on issues relating to payment policy and the design, implementation, and effectiveness of program integrity activities in Medicaid and the Children's Health Insurance Program (CHIP). Previously, Ms. Forbes served as director of the division of health and social service programs in the Office of Executive Program Information at the U.S. Department of Health and Human Services and as a vice president in the Medicaid practice at The Lewin Group. At Lewin, Ms. Forbes worked with every state Medicaid and CHIP program on issues relating to program integrity and eligibility quality control. She also has extensive experience with federal and state policy analysis, Medicaid program operations, and delivery system design. Ms. Forbes has a master of business administration from The George Washington University and a bachelor's degree in Russian and political science from Bryn Mawr College.

April Grady, M.P.Aff., is director of data development and analysis. In 2011, she was temporarily detailed to the Joint Select Committee on Deficit Reduction to provide Medicaid policy expertise during its deliberations. Prior to joining MACPAC, Ms. Grady worked at the Congressional Research Service and the Congressional Budget Office, where she provided non-partisan analyses of Medicaid, private health insurance, and other health policy issues. She has also held positions at the LBJ School of Public Affairs at The University of Texas at Austin and Mathematica Policy Research. Ms. Grady received a master of public affairs degree from the LBJ School of Public Affairs at The University of Texas and a bachelor of arts in policy studies from Syracuse University.

Benjamin Granata is a finance/budget specialist. His work focuses on reviewing financial documents to ensure completeness and accuracy for processing and recording in the financial systems. Mr. Granata graduated from Towson University with a bachelor's degree in business administration, specializing in project management.

Lindsay Hebert is a policy and research intern. Her work focuses on eligibility and benefits, particularly pertaining to the Affordable Care Act. Previously, she was a research assistant at The Johns Hopkins School of Medicine, focusing on patient safety initiatives in the department of pediatric oncology. Prior to that, she was a project coordinator in the Pediatric Intensive Care Unit at The Johns Hopkins Hospital. Ms. Hebert holds a bachelor of arts degree from the University of Florida and will receive a master of science in public health from The Johns Hopkins Bloomberg School of Public Health in May.

Angela Lello, M.P.Aff., is a senior analyst. Her work focuses on Medicaid for people with disabilities, particularly long-term services and supports (LTSS). Previously she was a Kennedy Public Policy Fellow at the U.S. Department of Health and Human Services (HHS), Administration on Intellectual and Developmental Disabilities, conducting policy research and analysis on a variety of HHS initiatives. Her prior work included analyzing and developing LTSS for people with disabilities while at the Texas Department of Aging and Disability Services and the Texas Council for Developmental Disabilities. Ms. Lello received a master of public affairs from the LBJ School of Public Affairs at The University of Texas.

Molly McGinn-Shapiro, M.P.P., is a senior analyst. Her work focuses on issues related to individuals dually eligible for Medicaid and Medicare. Previously, she was the special assistant to the executive vice president of the Henry J. Kaiser Family Foundation and to the executive director of the Kaiser Commission on Medicaid and the Uninsured. Ms. McGinn-Shapiro holds a master of public policy degree from Georgetown University's Georgetown Public Policy Institute.

Ellen O'Brien, Ph.D., is director of long-term services and supports. She was previously research associate professor at the Georgetown University Health Policy Institute and she has held positions at the AARP Public Policy Institute and in the U.S. Department of Health and Human Services (the Health Care Financing Administration—now the Centers for Medicare and Medicaid Services (CMS)—and the CMS Center for Consumer Information and Insurance Oversight). Dr. O'Brien received a master's degree in economics from the University of Iowa and a doctorate in economics from the University of Notre Dame.

Chris Park, M.S., is a senior analyst. His work focuses on issues related to managed care payment and Medicaid drug policy and provides data analyses using Medicaid administrative data. Prior to MACPAC, he was a senior consultant at The Lewin Group. At Lewin, he provided quantitative analyses and technical assistance on Medicaid policy issues, including Medicaid managed care capitation rate setting and pharmacy reimbursement and cost-containment initiatives. Mr. Park has a master of science degree in health policy and management from the Harvard School of Public Health and a bachelor of science degree in chemistry from the University of Virginia.

Chris Peterson, M.P.P., is director of eligibility, enrollment, and benefits. Prior to joining MACPAC, he was a specialist in health care financing at the Congressional Research Service, where he worked on major health legislation. Prior to that, he worked for the Agency for Healthcare Research and Quality and the National Bipartisan Commission on the Future of Medicare. Mr. Peterson has a master of public policy degree from Georgetown University's Georgetown Public Policy Institute and a bachelor of science degree in mathematics from Missouri Western State University.

Ken Pezzella is chief financial officer. He has more than 10 years of federal financial management and accounting experience in both the public and private sectors. Mr. Pezzella also has broad operations and business experience, and is a proud veteran of the U.S. Coast Guard.

Anne L. Schwartz, Ph.D., is executive director. Dr. Schwartz previously served as deputy editor at *Health Affairs*; vice president at Grantmakers In Health, a national organization providing strategic advice and educational programs for foundations and corporate giving programs working on health issues; and special assistant to the executive director and senior analyst at the Physician Payment Review Commission, a precursor to the Medicare Payment Advisory Commission. Earlier, she held positions on committee and personal staff for the U.S. House of Representatives. Dr. Schwartz earned a doctorate in health policy from the School of Hygiene and Public Health at The Johns Hopkins University.

Lois Simon, M.H.S., is director of managed care. Prior to joining MACPAC, she served as director of the Bureau of Program Planning and Implementation in the Division of Managed Care at the New York State Office of Health Insurance Programs and was director of compliance at HIP Health Plan of New York (now EmblemHealth) where she was instrumental in the implementation of the plan's compliance program, the Health Insurance Portability and Accountability Act (HIPAA), and disaster recovery efforts. Ms. Simon has also held positions with the Commonwealth Fund and the Kaiser Commission on the Future of Medicaid (now the Kaiser Commission on Medicaid and the Uninsured). She began her career working in the Congressional Budget Office and in the office of U.S. Representative Joseph P. Addabbo. Ms. Simon received her master of health science degree from the School of Hygiene and Public Health at The Johns Hopkins University.

Anna Sommers, Ph.D., M.P.Aff., M.S., is director of access and quality. Dr. Sommers has conducted health services research related to Medicaid programs for over 15 years. Previously, she was a senior health researcher at the Center for Studying Health System Change in Washington, D.C. Prior to that, she was a senior research analyst at The Hilltop Institute, University of Maryland, Baltimore County, and a research associate at the Urban Institute. Dr. Sommers received a doctorate and master of science in health services research, policy and administration from the University of Minnesota School of Public Health, and a master of public affairs degree from the University of Minnesota's Hubert H. Humphrey Institute of Public Affairs.

Mary Ellen Stahlman, M.H.S.A., is senior advisor for congressional affairs. In addition to managing MACPAC's congressional affairs, she assists in directing MACPAC's policy agenda and editing and producing the Commission's reports to the Congress. Previously, she held positions at the National Health Policy Forum, focusing on Medicare issues including private plans and the Medicare drug benefit. She served at the Centers for Medicare & Medicaid Services and its predecessor agency—the Health Care Financing Administration—for 18 years, including as deputy director of policy. Ms. Stahlman received a master of health services administration from The George Washington University and a bachelor of arts from Bates College.

James Teisl, M.P.H., is a principal analyst focused on issues related to Medicaid payment and financing. Previously, he was a senior consultant with The Lewin Group and has also worked for the Greater New York Hospital Association and the Ohio Medicaid program. Mr. Teisl received a master of public health from The Johns Hopkins Bloomberg School of Public Health.

Ricardo Villeta, M.B.A., is deputy director of operations, finance, and management with overall responsibility for management of the MACPAC budget and resources. Mr. Villeta directs all operations related to financial management and budget, procurement, human resources, information technology, and contracting. Previously, he was the senior vice president and chief management officer for the Academy for Educational Development, a private, non-profit educational organization which provided training, education and technical assistance throughout the United States and in more than 50 countries. Mr. Villeta holds a master of business administration degree from The George Washington University and a bachelor of science degree from Georgetown University.

Eileen Wilkie is the administrative officer and is responsible for human resources, office maintenance, and coordinating travel and Commission meetings. Previously, she held similar roles at National Public Radio and the National Endowment for Democracy. Ms. Wilkie has a bachelor of science in political science from the University of Notre Dame.

www.ingramcontent.com/pod-product-compliance
Lightning Source LLC
Chambersburg PA
CBHW081723170526
45167CB00009B/3677